sex tips for girls

sex tips for girls

First published 2002 by Channel 4 Books
an imprint of Pan Macmillan Ltd
20 New Wharf Road, London N1 9RR
Basingstoke and Oxford
Associated companies throughout the world
www.panmacmillan.com

ISBN 0 7522 6510 5

3 5 7 9 8 6 4

A CIP catalogue record for this book is available from the British Library.

Designed and typeset by seagulls

Printed by Mackays of Chatham plc

RICOCHET
south

This book accompanies the television series *Sex Tips for Girls*
and *More Sex Tips for Girls*, made by Ricochet South for Channel 4.

Executive Producers: Nick Powell, Amanda Murphy
Series Producer: Izzie Pick

Flic Everett would like to thank Lou Paget and Anne Hooper.

www.loupaget.com
Lou Paget is an international best-selling author and sex educator.

www.annehooper.com
Anne Hooper is a sexual and marital therapist and best-selling author
of *Ultimate Sex Guide*, *Anne Hooper's Kama Sutra* and *Sex Tips*.

contents

introduction

Sex can be the greatest event in the world. It can also be less fun than turning up to the circus a week late, and finding only a patch of flattened grass where you were expecting a three-ring extravaganza. Yet there's so much written, spoken and discussed when it comes to sex, you'd think we should all be sexperts, tweaking nipples in our sleep, and bringing partners to dizzy orgasm with one hand whilst polishing our tool-kit of vibrators with the other.

The truth is, though, sex is never that simple – how much you enjoy it depends on a huge number of factors, from who you're doing it with, to how tired you are, whether the bed (or wheelbarrow) squeaks, and how you're feeling about yourself. Far too much sex advice is aimed at people who don't appear to be living a real sex life at all – they're simply mating on some strange style-planet where emotions don't count, and everyone's a master of yoga. *Sex Tips for Girls*, however, is all about real people, with normal sex lives.

Sometimes we want a ten-course banquet of physical delights, other times sexual fast food is all that's required. Real sex is funny, enjoyable, occasionally silly, and when you're with the right person, can include everything from a reassuring cuddle to an epic journey of discovery.

And what real people having real sex need most are a few pointers to make sure all types of sex are as enjoyable as they possibly can be. All the tips in *Sex Tips for Girls* have been tried and tested by real couples – and not the weird 'real couples' you hear about who've been plucked straight from Soho vice dens, either. There are experts who truly know what they're talking about to help out, too, and not one of them suggests that swinging naked from a chandelier is a valid or even erotic way to pass the time. We don't have drawings, of course – but if we did, rest assured that none of them would feature men with beards that eagles could happily nest in.

So if you want to feel inadequate, confused, and worried that your sex life is uselessly dull and hopeless, go buy another sex manual. If, however, you want a whole lot of practical tips, clear explanations, and enjoyable experiences … then go right ahead and read on.

1 foreplay

If there's anyone who doesn't know by now that foreplay is generally necessary for good sex, they've almost certainly been living in some *Jurassic* swamp, practising their hot moves on the last remaining diplodocus. Having said that, while most men and women are eager enough to rev up their partners with some hand and tongue action, plenty of them are still a little unsure, and approach the whole thing as if they're constructing some *Blue Peter*-style origami swan, complete with fiddly flaps and bits that won't stick down. Foreplay is, simply, the art of turning your partner on enough to make them want to have sex – though it can be enjoyable as an experience in its own right, of course.

For men, that might be simply a case of 'Fancy a shag?', though even the most hair-trigger man will still appreciate having his penis handled delicately first. And for women, it's a far lengthier process, involving chat, jokes, stroking, cuddling, licking, nibbling and squeezing. Unless, of course, she's already desperate for it – and even then, you need to devote a good half-hour to her bodily needs first.

Foreplay begins, as they say, 'outside the bedroom'. We're not going to bother with all the 'it begins with a mental connection' stuff, though, because the assumption is that if you're about to get naked you already have some kind of connection going on, even if it's only one akin to two dodgy electric wires twisted together.

Foreplay isn't just about manipulating each other's genitals to an explosive point of no return, it's about touching, stroking and caressing each other before you even head below the waistline. Women's bodies are programmed to respond to the softest, most featherlike of touches, and sometimes the merest brush of lips on neck can result in feelings of orgasmic intensity. Men can be a little more claylike in their responses, and may need a firmer hand applied to their erogenous zones – but that doesn't mean they can't appreciate gentle caresses, or being softly stroked, in the manner of a startled horse. It is possible to get in the mood for sex before you even see each other though – by talking dirty.

talking dirty

Foreplay isn't just about physical frolicking – it's about getting into the mood for sex, and while for some men that means a quick scrub with soap on a rope and a brief thought about Sarah Michelle Gellar in a corset, for women it's a little more complex than that. Which is where talking dirty comes in. Given that sex is at least as much down to mental stimulation as

---

TIP

An easy way to get into talking dirty if you find it a little difficult at first is to use words normally associated with food ('boil me now … put me on a slow roast and turn me halfway through' – no, I'm joking). Words like eat, lick, suck, taste, and nibble are useful. And using the blunt, Anglo-Saxon words for acts is better than the medical terms – 'vagina' sounds like you're a doctor about to perform an examination, whereas 'cunt' is suitably earthy and basic. But don't get too hung up on the Anglo-Saxon stuff, you don't want to be wondering what the Middle English for 'clitoris' is at the crucial moment.

Dirty talk doesn't have to be terribly articulate. If the problem is that you worry you'll lose the thread halfway through, don't – he really won't care. Even a few phrases thrown in here and there will do the job – 'fuck me hard' doesn't require any great mental powers. To begin with, get three dice, and write six adjectives on one – such as 'hot', 'sexy', 'wet' and so on. Then on the second, write six verbs – 'fuck', 'touch', 'thrust' – and on the final one, write six nouns. Then throw the dice, and all you need to come up with are the joining-up words – and say them out loud.

physical –well, good sex is, crap sex is generally down to eight pints – it pays to rev up the engine before attempting to drive the car, as it were. So 'nice tits, get your keks off' probably won't do it, but a little more sophisticated dirty talk just might.

You can e-mail your partner during the day, and state a few things you might like to do to them later – but it helps if they're between meetings, not actually in one. Typing 'I want your hot cock inside me,' just as the boss is standing behind him waiting for him to download the quarterly figures, is not sexy, it's just daft. But once you've ensured he's free to communicate, go right ahead and be as rude as possible.

Text messages are an equally sexy way of getting your message across – though make sure you don't become such an expert at teen-style text language that he has absolutely no idea what you're talking about. A quick 'I want u 2 cum on my tits,' however, should leave him in no doubt about your intentions. And hopefully, his colleague hasn't borrowed his phone for the afternoon.

TIP

Because men are so visual, if you are going to e-mail or text him with wild promises of things you're going to do to him, explain properly so he can get the picture. Instead of saying 'have surprise 4 u later,' say 'will give u blow job on way home frm wrk,' for example. Though if your journey home involves a packed commuter train, maybe then isn't the time ... Equally, when he mails you he shouldn't make demands, he should simply outline what he'd like to do to you. Of course, he may well get a blow job, but telling you he'll go down on you for hours will be a more appealing text message, right?

Phone sex is another way of getting yourselves hot, by talking each other to the point of orgasm – 'now I'm touching your hard cock ... now I'm sliding my hand up and down it ...' style of chit-chat should work. Of course, he has to reciprocate, and tell you how much he wants to be inside your beautiful cunt, fucking you senseless ... With talking dirty, never forget, however, that it's only a short step from 'huge turn-on' to 'sounding stupid'. Anything that veers too much towards porn-star small talk is never going to work. So 'ride my tool, bitch' will simply sound silly, as will 'fill my tunnel with your hot cum' – unless it happens to work for you, in which case go ahead, and good luck with finding a distributor.

Find a language that is intimate and sexual for you, whether that's 'Poppa's baby rabbit want his big carrot' (if it is, take yourself away, you odd-ball) or simply 'I want you in me, right now.' If you're too shy for dirty fore-play-talk, then texting and e-mailing are godsends. Don't ignore their potential, will you?

little kisses

Obviously, kissing is an element of foreplay. But most of us mastered the basic snog manoeuvre by the fourth year of Big School, so we'll assume you know pretty much what you should be doing with your tongue by now, at least when it happens to be in someone else's mouth. It's what to do with it when it's anywhere else on his body that matters when it comes to foreplay.

And while most sex manuals suggest you should 'lick him all over', that's just going to make him feel like a giant kitten. That can work for certain weird types in furry body suits, but for the average guy, a full lick-bath will just leave him feeling like he should be scratching for fleas and chasing wool while he's at it. The tongue should be used sparingly, but effectively – like garlic in pasta dishes. A little can make all the difference, but too much is just unpleasant.

Start with a delicate trail along the side of his neck, just below his ear – you may want to swirl it into the hollow crevice of his shoulder-blade

---

TIP

Shaving your pubes can be a thrill for both of you – shaving his will immediately make his penis look bigger, while shaving yours is sexy because it exposes more of your labia. It also means that when you have sex, there's more friction, and your clitoris gets more effectively ground into. Shaving, however, is incredibly itchy when it grows back, so depilating is a more attractive option – and also makes it easier to trim neatly, particularly if your hair tends to be quite bushy. If shaving is a turn-on for you, then shave each other – but only when you're sober, alright?

too, which will activate a whole bunch of tiny nerves. Alternate this with tiny, brushing kisses — few guys want their shoulder snogged, but there's a big difference between that and light stimulation of the skin. The back of his neck is another hotspot, which will respond with great alacrity to a little tongue-flicking, particularly if you move down to the top of his spine and swirl the tip (of your tongue, not his spine, silly) in small circles.

Most men don't like having their faces licked — back to kittens — but a little kissing and licking of the nipples is a very fine thing. Learn from men's mistakes, and don't twiddle them like you're tuning into a Mexican pirate station. A light swish of the tongue, back and forth, across them, or a little gentle sucking, should be enough to fire up the connection to his penis almost instantly. If he isn't in touch with the Power of Nipple, he's probably got all sorts of hang-ups about it being 'womanly' or somesuch, so it's your job to put him straight, and explain that god gave men nipples for a reason, and it clearly wasn't to feed babies.

If you're inclined, you can kiss and lick his feet, but I can think of about

---

TIP

If you're going to take control in bed and initiate sex, you have to be able to state what you want. A men's magazine survey found that the most common response from women when asked what they want by their partners is 'I don't mind,' or 'whatever you feel like'. You bloody do mind, you're just too shy to tell him so. Practice by saying 'that feels great,' or 'mm, that's lovely,' then when he asks you can at least say 'I loved that thing you were doing when I said it felt amazing'. Otherwise you'll both be left unsatisfied — so pick up on his cues too.

fifty things to do that might be more fun, starting with 'make a *papier maché* model of Hong Kong' and ending with 'arrange a series of woodlice in order of size'. Still, if it works for you, you go girlfriend, and suck those toes. Of course, if you expect him to suck yours, you may have to reciprocate, though you may wish to point out that your feet are probably quite fragrant and your toenails are polished a lovely pink shade, unlike the scaly yellow monstrosities that are most men's extremities.

So restrain your licking and nibbly kissing to his inner thighs – because if they're yellow and scaly, then Houston, you have a problem. The worst thing about them should be the hairs that get caught in your teeth. Aside from that, inner thighs are a source of great wonder and delight – they are packed with nerve endings, just waiting to be stimulated, with a direct connection to the genitalia. Just lick and kiss your way up them, stopping just short of the boxer-short line (whether he's wearing them or not), to have him writhing with desire. This works just as well, if not better, for you too, of course – he should use his hand to stroke one thigh whilst kissing and trailing his tongue up the inside of the other. Bottoms respond to kissing beautifully, too – we're not talking about the inner workings at this point, that's a whole other chapter – but the buttocks themselves only require

Using little brushes on each other's skin feels like being touched all over by delicate fingertips – and therefore, great. Get a little selection of artists' paintbrushes, feather dusters, ostrich feathers and the like, and try them out on each others' skin, moving from fairly hard bristles (no, not a scrubbing brush) down to the tip of a feather to see what works best. There are so many nerves in the skin that just being touched with a soft brush can be a deeply erotic experience.

the lightest touch to spring into life. Kiss the hollow at the bottom of the back, and run your tongue in circles over his bum – unless it's spotty, in which case you are officially exempt from all bum-related duties. He should kiss yours too, and can even try the odd, gentle, bite – we're not talking about him sinking his teeth in like it's a club sandwich, though.

If you want to, you can try the full kiss and lick experience on each others' hands, but it's a bit too similar to a whole knights-about-to-joust scenario, as he kisses your lily-white hand, and licks your wrist. Actually, that's just weird. Save it for the ears – perhaps the part of the body that responds most effectively to kissing and nibbling. Be very careful, however, to do this quietly, or it'll sound like someone with a harelip eating crisps in your ear canal.

If you're short of time, though, have a lot of kissing and licking to deposit, and aren't sure where to head for, then go straight to the erogenous zones without passing 'Go'. They are buttocks, breasts (or nipples for men, obviously), neck and lips. Some individuals may have urgently erotic elbows, but it's rare – so stick with what you know. And never lick like a mummy cat trying to dislodge a recalcitrant flea.

massage

If licking all over sounds like a whole lot of effort, then offer a massage instead. Massage is not just for sports stars and dodgy men at 'Cleopatra's Body Temple, all new staff ...' It is in fact the perfect way to turn each other on, relax muscles that are knotted more tightly than oak tree roots, and get as close as you can to orgasm without actually having one. A really good massage should leave your whole body feeling flooded with sensual delight, with all your dormant nerve-endings waking up like Rip Van Winkle after a hundred-year nap. You can choose just to massage a small area – shoulders, bum, penis – or go for the full body meltdown-massage, which should take at least an hour if you're doing it right. A few brisk jiggles of the shoulders does not count as doing it right, incidentally.

how to give a sexy massage

He (or you) should lie on your front – that way you're not going to be distracted by his bobbing erection every time you glance down. Cover your hands in scented massage oil and then warm them. Begin at the neck, by placing your hands on either side and stroking lightly upwards just under his ears. Then move your thumbs down to the top of his spine, and rub in small circles, without pressing too hard – remember you aren't dealing with sporting injuries, merely trying to activate erotic rushes of feeling. Move right down his spine, pressing and moulding with your thumbs, and when you reach the bottom, sweep your hands across his buttocks. Never taking your hands off his skin, sweep your palms back up again, then work your thumbs just under his shoulder blades to gently push away tension. Once you've dealt with any basic knots, you can get flirtier – if you have long nails, scrape them (lightly, we're not onto S&M yet) across his back, and run them down his spine, or use them to stroke patterns on his skin. If not, just use your fingertips to caress the sides of his body – a horribly neglected area – and trail along his spine. If you really want to give him a sensual massage, finish off by covering your breasts in oil, and lying on his back, rubbing yourself up and down. Of course, he'll want to turn over immediately and have sex with you, but don't let him – it's all about arousing him slowly.

If you're dying for a turn yourself, stop at this point – but if you're going for the full effect, now's the time to give his bum a good kneading. Just take a buttock in each hand, and squeeze and release as if you're making a particularly tasty loaf, then work your way down to the tops of his thighs, where you turn your fingers inwards, and continue to massage his inner thighs, going as close as you dare – gently – to his balls. Work up and down, and if you want to you can move onto his calves, but if so, be aware that a calf massage is a little too physiotherapist-friendly to be truly erotic. A foot massage can be arousing, too, but for many, feet are the work of the devil, and best avoided, however attractive the legs attached to them

---

TIP

When you're giving a massage, you should both be naked. It's no fun if only one of you is playing. Straddle his bum, and lean on your hands so your weight is mainly on his upper back, and use it as leverage to place the pressure of your hands on his shoulder-blades. The back massage feels nice, but the thing that really matters is whether you've got your bits grinding into his buttocks as you massage. If so, his muscular tensions will be dissipated in a matter of minutes, I'm sure – particularly if you then suggest a full frontal massage, and adopt the same straddling position for this one, too.

> **TIP**
>
> When he's massaging you, allow him to give you a genital massage. This isn't simply a matter of placing his hand over your genitals and rubbing away – though that can be nice. A proper labial massage involves a technique known as 'wibbling' – sounds stupid; feels great. And you can call it Arthur if you want, it still feels good. He should use his fingers to gently pull and release all the way up and down each side of the labia. I said 'gently'. He can go as far as the clitoris, then go back down the other side, without removing his hands at all – and without actually touching your clit – to drive you wild with anticipation.

---

may be. If you don't fear feet, though, use the ball of your thumb to rub gently around the edge of the foot, and work your way into the middle, pressing lightly. According to reflexologists, each part corresponds to a different part of the body, so if your partner suddenly gets a terrible pain in their liver, you're probably being too rough. Firm enough not to tickle, not so firm that they're in agony is the basic rule of massage – and that counts for everywhere.

Of course, you can massage the genitals, too – but even touching them is a whole new, er, ballgame, and instantly moves your massage on from 'innocently pleasurable' to 'downright thrilling'.

touching breasts

Touching breasts is simple. Just treat them gently, never pull, poke, tug or jiggle them – they are not beanbags handed out to kindergarten children, they are sensitive organs in their own right that must be treated with respect. Respectful treatment can include stroking the whole breast area, caressing it with the fingertips, gradually drawing closer to the nipple, which will be rubbed between thumb and forefinger, or lightly tweaked, or stroked. It should not, however, be twiddled, flicked, pulled or pressed, because try as he might, he will never get Jazz FM on your breasts.

The tongue is a very useful addition to breast-fondling – he should use it to lick delicately across your breasts and shoulders, and finally activate your nipples by flicking it across them, or circling it on them. Nipples can be sucked, gently – if he does it too hard, all sorts of comedy noises might ensue – and they can also be licked very successfully. Breasts are simple – think gentle and he can't go too badly wrong.

touching the bits

This is where it starts to get complicated. Because the genitals are a mass of nerve-endings more tangled and complex than an electricity substation, if you're going to stimulate them, it has to be done correctly, or you will

---

TIP

It seems obvious as sex tips go – but that doesn't make it less valid. A huge number of grown women have no idea what their bits look like. So in order to get a good look and stand any chance of finding the relevant areas when you're masturbating, it's a very good idea to get a hand mirror and a decent light, and have a look. Once you know where your clitoris and vagina are and what they look like, it's much easier to touch yourself in a way that works – and to teach him to do the same.

TIP

A handy way to get yourself in the mood for sex quickly and easily is to focus on a sexy memory. Close your eyes and fully experience it again – how it felt, what you thought at the time, what it looked like … often the day after an intense sexual experience, you're raring to go again because the memory is so fresh, you're still turned on. By reconnecting with that memory, you'll feel that wave of lust all over again – and hey, so what if it was with an ex-boyfriend? It's not like you need to tell him what you're thinking about, is it?

---

simply cause pain and annoyance. Many a bloke has assumed his girlfriend's writhing in ecstasy when she is, in fact, simply attempting to get away from his ham-fisted attempts at masturbating her. It shouldn't be that difficult but, in truth, sadly, it is. Even the penis, which many women assume is an idiot-proof device, can be handled wrongly. Treating each other's genitals like baby toys – pulling, prodding, violent jiggling and the like – is a profoundly bad idea. Think of yourself as Aladdin holding the magic lamp – you have to rub in exactly the right way to unleash the orgasm-genie. Though if he's wearing pants that actually say 'rub gently and a genie will appear' on the front, you don't have to do anything except catch the next plane out of town.

handling her bits

Make him memorise this section so well that he can recite it backwards on demand. Because only then can you be sure that he actually knows what he's doing. For men, the old 'what's a clitoris?' dark ages are largely over, but just because they know what one is and where it is – well, most do, but for those who missed out on remedial biology class, it's the little tiny pea-shaped thing tucked inside her labia, at the point where her legs join together – doesn't mean that they know what to do with it. Some believe a steady, grinding pressure is required. Others flick it around like it's a pin-ball flipper. Still others approach it like a dangerous insect, essaying a little tap, then retreating in terror. All of these methods are basically hopeless. Never mind whether she orgasms or not, she's not even going to get to the first level of enjoyment with this kind of action.

The first rule of clitoral stimulation, then, is lubrication. To put it bluntly, he's never going to get anywhere attempting to rub a dry clitoris. If she isn't wet enough – and women only get wet when they're thoroughly turned on – then he has to use an artificial lubricant such as KY Jelly. This has the effect of allowing his fingers to slide back and forth without any painful friction – and tragically, many men are still unaware that their attempts at clitoris-based passion are simply agonising, because they didn't make sure it was wet enough before they galloped in with their rough fingers. The clitoris is the single most sensitive part of a woman (if you

TIP

Men should never use the 'dip test' to check whether you're wet enough to have sex – you know, the one where he twiddles your nipples, snogs you a bit, then thrusts his hand into your knickers and prods his finger in the direction of your vagina, to see if you're even slightly lubricated. It's not a terribly classy way to find out – so if he is venturing down there, it's polite to stay and actually stimulate your clitoris. That way, you almost certainly will be ready by the time he wants to go any further.

Women tend to be much more inhibited about their bodies than men are, and consequently you find it harder to let go and enjoy sex, because you're worrying what your bum looks like, or thinking your stomach's hanging down. Two things – build up your own confidence by dimming the lights, lighting candles, wearing your sexiest clothes or underwear, and more importantly, try to accept that he really does fancy you and he really isn't looking at your stretch-marks. Because he's just glad to be there.

discount her feelings regarding the size of her arse) and must be treated as if you're buffing up a precious jewel, rather than the army boot-polishing antics that many men favour. So before you do anything else, lubricate – a pea-sized amount is enough. If you have no KY to hand, saliva is better than nothing, but try not to make hawking noises like a 13-year-old lad at a bus stop. Just lick your finger, OK?

Once you've located the clitoris, make small circles around it with your fingertip, or two fingertips. You'll be able to tell if you're doing it right because she will make noises of appreciation. If you're doing it wrong, she'll catch her breath and bite her lip and look pained. How hard can it be to tell? You can either go straight for her orgasm, without passing go, by maintaining a steady rhythm, building up the speed slightly as she starts to gasp, or you can take the scenic bus route, and begin by stroking her pubic hair, then stroke her outer labia, before pressing more firmly and reaching her inner parts – you can circle your finger around her vagina, and push it in a little way, remembering that only the first 3 inches have nerve-endings. You're unlikely to reach the G-spot with your finger – it's a

> **TIP**
>
> Saliva is a very useful lubricant, but only in the absence of anything else. If you can, buy a manufactured one such as KY Jelly or Probe (mmm!), because they're properly formulated to replicate vaginal lubrication, and feel much nicer – plus they don't immediately dry, which saliva does. Even if you have no trouble producing your own lubrication, it helps to have some for hand jobs, or very lengthy sex sessions – and make sure it's water-based, as oil-based products can rot condoms.

little like trying to locate buried treasure in an underground cave without a flashlight – but if you have long fingers, you should curve one over the front wall of the vagina, and feel around for a little spongy pad. That's the G-spot, and when stimulated it may or may not produce a spectacular orgasm. If not, don't worry, it's perfectly alright. Some women like their clitoris played with while you have a finger or two inside them, but most will never come through vaginal stimulation alone, however hard you thrust your fingers in and out. Some even like to have a finger on or up their anus, one in the vagina, and the rest dancing around on the clitoris – but it takes a dextrous man to achieve that one without getting hand-cramp.

The basic clitoral orgasm, though, is often best achieved through accompanying nipple-stimulation. If you can tweak one with the other hand, and contrive to move you head round so you're licking the other, she may need scraping off the ceiling with a palette-knife when she comes. Coming round the mountain has nothing on this one. If she merely finds three-point excitement confusing though, stick with what you know, and keep up a gentle but steady pressure around her clitoris.

You can cup your whole hand over her pubic bone, fingers upwards, and rub her slowly with the heel of it for a different kind of stimulation – but you can get more precision-work in with fingertips. When she does come, take your hand away – there's nothing worse than a suddenly-sensitive clitoris subjected to pressure, and she does not need a final, flourishing rub to finish with – she just needs to recover for a few minutes, till the sensitivity subsides back to normal levels. It's generally better to let her come before sex if she isn't a woman who comes through intercourse – otherwise she'll be sitting up in bed like a meerkat , waiting for her turn, and you'll be a spent, exhausted husk drifting into a coma on the other side of the bed.

touching his bits

Giving a hand job is a little like polishing a wooden banister to a gleaming shine. It's hard work, but ultimately satisfying. It's all about the grip you use – there's no immediate need for fancy techniques, though they can be highly entertaining for him – but as long as you're holding it right, he's going to come either way. Even if the house is surrounded with police vans and officers shouting through megaphones, he'll still have an orgasm before he goes out with his hands up.

the basic hand job that works – every time

To give a great hand job, you don't actually need lubrication, but it doesn't hurt – it also has the added bonus of feeling a little more like a blow job for him that way. So if you do use it, a blob the size of a penny should do the trick, and allow your hand to slide more easily up and down his shaft. Although women like to be caressed in other areas before he heads for her bits, for men, the whole 'creeping up on you gently' idea is somewhat less important. In fact, most men are likely to be attempting to nudge your hand downwards shortly after 'hello'. So if you do want to go more slowly, just kiss him, stroke his nipples, knead his bum, and then get down there before he expires through need.

It sounds obvious, but if you're right-handed, use your right hand, otherwise your weaker arm will begin to seize up about thirty seconds before he comes. He'll be gasping and panting like Ivor the Engine going up Snowdon, and you'll be muttering 'I can't go on, really sorry …' as your wrist goes floppy with exertion.

Make sure you're lying comfortably so you don't have to rearrange yourself halfway through – this is particularly important if he's touching you at the same time, of course. Now, grasp his penis with your whole hand. Too many women make the mistake of balancing it as if it was a china teacup, between finger and thumb. This may eventually make him orgasm,

---

TIP

If he's desperate for a shag and you just want to go to sleep, it really is a kindness to offer a hand job – it's the least trouble for you, and he'll be happy and grateful. The fast-results hand job is simply a matter of exposing your breasts so he's got something to look at, lubricating your hand with KY, and starting fast. Forget the gradual build-up, just get a rhythm going, then go hell for leather, swapping hands seamlessly like a drummer if your arm starts to seize up before he comes. It really shouldn't take more than three minutes – put the radio on, it's the length of a song, and perhaps 'Show Me Heaven' will be playing.

TIP

When you're giving him a hand job and he starts to come, don't automatically speed up. If you go against that instinct, and carry on rubbing slowly – about one stroke a second, instead of the average three a second that orgasm normally encourages – it will deepen and prolong his orgasm. He'll still come, but it will be a much slower sensation. Obviously, he'll be throwing himself around, trying to get you to speed up, so it may be worth explaining your cunning plan to him first, and seeing whether it works for him.

---

but it will take a couple of days. You need to wrap your fingers round it with your thumb at the top, encircling the head, so just enough is poking out to enable you to rub up and down freely. Your fingers should be curved round back towards yourself, so the whole shaft is enclosed in your fist. Grip as though you mean it, but not hard enough to cut off his blood supply. A penis can take a lot more pressure than a clitoris, so don't be afraid to be firm.

Begin with a steady pace, making sure the foreskin pulls up over the head, and rolls back without impediment – if he's circumcised, you may need more lubrication. As he gets more excited (in about three seconds, usually), speed up your pace as if you're polishing that banister and the master of the house is walking down the hall towards you, about to check it for reflective sheen. Just as you get so fast you know your arm can't take the pain, he will almost certainly come – try to angle his penis so it goes all over his chest, rather than your hair.

And obviously, be careful, in your excitement, not to wrench it wildly to the side. (I won't go into the potential consequences, but suffice it to

Another suggestion for a memorable hand job – the 'countdown' stroke – does not involve trying to make a new word out of the letters 'p-e-n-i-s e-x-t-e-n-s-i-o-n,' or conjuring up a vision of Richard Whitely to spur you on (please god, no). It is simply counting down hand strokes – with lubrication, give his penis nine strokes down, then nine up, followed by eight down, eight up, seven up ... yes, well, you get the idea, right down to zero. After which, you can shout 'blast off!' and proceed to do something even more explosive, whether that's a blow job or sex in the wheelbarrow position ... this stroke gets him right in the mood for it, and thoroughly builds up his excitement.

say they end up on the kind of e-mail attachment that bored lads send to their office-bound friends. Not pretty.)

To enhance the experience – not that it really needs it – some men like to have their balls stroked or, ideally, sucked, while you rub his penis. Make sure you can cope with multi-tasking though, otherwise it's like rubbing your tummy and patting your head, and can result in utter confusion all round. If that's too much like trouble, then suck or stroke his nipples as you go, or kiss his neck. As you approach the home straight, and if your guy is the liberal sort, you can slide a finger into his anus because this will stimulate his prostate gland and result in a madly intense orgasm for him. Afterwards he may say 'bloody hell, what was your finger doing up my bum?' But by then, he'll be more than aware of the positive benefits of doing such a thing.

If you want to caress his penis in a teasing fashion before you actually perform the full hand job experience, you need to focus on the frenulum – this is the tiny bit of skin that connects the head to the shaft, and responds well to very gentle stroking. Circle your fingers on the tip, then run them along the shaft, alongside the vein that runs up the front of his erect penis. Pay attention to his balls – never squeeze them, think of them as baby breasts, and treat them as you would wish your own breasts to be treated. Unless you get off on the idea of having them bitten really hard, of course.

Don't ignore the perineum – this is the bit of skin that connects his balls and his arse, and in itself connects to the prostate gland – so light pressure on this area will, again, intensify the sensations he's feeling. That would be 'light' pressure, however – don't get overexcited and start beeping away at it like it's a car-horn, whatever you do.

advanced technique

For those who mastered the basic hand job years ago, there are certain techniques that can enhance the whole thing – as taught by Lou Paget, Californian sex educator and best-selling author, and queen of the hot move. They may take a little practice to perfect – Lou likes to allow her subjects to work on a lifelike latex penis, but you may be reduced to trying out your moves on a large courgette, if you're unsure about the real thing. Still, once mastered it's like riding a bike – you'll never forget them.

the basketweave

Link your fingers together, so both hands are clasped around his shaft – you need lubrication for this, it makes the whole thing ten times easier – then push both hands down to the bottom of his shaft, twist them, and come back up, twist at the top, go back down. As he approaches orgasm, you can get less sophisticated. But grown men may well buy you diamonds for your ability to perform this manoeuvre.

the heartbeat

Again, clasp your hands – but this time, as you go up and then down the shaft, 'pulse' your hands in and out by squeezing lightly moving up or down the shaft without rotating. This will mimic the sensation of you tightening around him when he is inside you. He's unlikely to come this way, but who cares when it feels so nice?

the figure eight

One-handed, perform the basic hand job, but when you reach the top and bottom, give a gentle twist each time. This activates the nerve endings of his penis that wouldn't normally get a look in – and it's easy to do, which is a bonus.

2 positions

Having sex is easy. But having sex so you want to keep doing it with the same person is a little more difficult. While some of that may be down to how they look, and whether they smell of Givenchy Pour Homme or an overflowing ashtray, an awful lot is down to the position you choose to have sex in. There's something to be said for missionary, but sadly, that something is likely to be 'effective but dull.' Which means that for genuinely good sex, you need a repertoire of different positions, all of which will result in a happy sexual experience.

I could tell you all sorts about the Congress of the Water Buffalo, or how to make love hanging upside down from a rope, but it wouldn't be that much fun to actually put into practice. The Polaroids would be amazing, but the experience itself would definitely come under 'once only.' So the first basic question when it comes to finding a new and interesting sexual position is 'is it comfortable?' and the second basic question is 'is it enjoyable?' Only when the answer to both questions is 'yes' should you proceed.

Of, course, it's perfectly possible to have enjoyable and orgasmic sex without throwing each other around like Russian shot-putters, but the roll-on roll-off ferry position is frankly in danger of becoming dull after a few years' repetition. There are over a hundred positions that it's actually possible to contort yourself into – but the real question is, why would you want to? If it's not working for one of you, it's a dud. So while he may be having just the best time ever with your legs behind your ears and your

A useful sexual position, though it sounds appalling, is The Clamp. You lie in the standard missionary position, then while he penetrates you, bring your legs together so the base of his penis is trapped between your thighs, and his legs are straddling yours for a change. This significantly increases the amount of friction his penis can feel, while your clitoris benefits from the extra pressure too. The difficulty is, he's more likely to fall out while thrusting, and there's nothing more painful than a mis-thrust penis. Still, it's worth doing now and then, if only for the novelty value of swapping your usual leg-positions around.

head wedged between his thighs, if you feel like a human pretzel, orgasm will be a distant dream.

positions that work

Certain basic (and not so basic) positions will always offer a good time. Once you have them in your armoury, sex becomes a far more enticing prospect, because you automatically know what's going to give your clitoris the best pressure, or where you need to put your legs to activate your G-spot. Forget the *Kama Sutra*, it may have had some decent pictures if you were a love-starved ancient, but for today's couple, trying to arrange yourselves into anything similar is like trying to assemble flat-pack furniture in the dark without a screwdriver.

There are, however, a few positions that work for almost everybody, regardless of yogic ability. The most popular – assuming anybody tells the truth in sex surveys – are woman on top, and missionary. But as we're trying to make life more exciting, we'll leave missionary till later, and concentrate on The Ten Positions That Always Work. At least they do unless you've just had a row, developed a migraine, or recently been for back surgery.

the ten positions that always work

spoons

The Spoons position is the easiest and simplest of all sexual positions. All you do is lie on your side, with him behind you. He shunts up so his willy is aligned with your bits, like a spaceship docking – it helps if you both bend your legs and tuck into each other, with his arm round your waist, so his hand can cup your breast. His other arm can lie along your back, or form a pillow for your head. Push your bum into his groin until your bits are properly aligned – then in it goes. Leverage for thrusting is provided by the fact that he's holding your waist. This is a handy position for stimulating the front wall of your vagina, where the elusive G-spot may reside. It's not so good for your clitoris – unless before entering, he uses his penis tip to masturbate you, whilst you clamp it between your thighs, ensuring that he has an equally good time.

scissors

Easier to perform than describe, the Scissors manoeuvre starts with you lying side by side, facing each other. Now listen carefully. You put one leg over his outer hip, and he grabs your bum. This enables him to penetrate you effectively, while you use your leg as a lever to help him thrust. He can also lick your breasts (or if he's of a mind to, he can stick his head between them and go 'bbbbbbffflllbb', but you may not want him to, of course). You need to keep your underneath leg pressed against his, while your top arm goes round his waist. Look, it's really not that complicated, but feel free to practise with dolls first, of course. The bonus here is that his groin rubs your clitoral area, and you can kiss. It's also perfect placement for getting a finger up his bum, just before he comes. Though that may be a little too graphic for dolly.

doggy

Ask any man his favourite position for a full-on sex-fest shag, as opposed to the lovey-dovey romantic kind, and if he doesn't say 'doggy', he's almost certainly lying. This is possibly the sexiest position ever invented, but sadly, some women feel it's a little demeaning. It is, if he's behind you snarling 'I don't wanna see your face bitch, I just want you to bark'. But assuming he isn't,

---

TIP

Men are visual wee creatures, so actually seeing you while you're having sex is fairly high up his wish-list. But even better is watching himself have sex – with you, naturally. The best sex to watch in front of a mirror is either doggy style or standing up, both of which enable you to twist your heads to look, or give you the chance to do it with you both facing the mirror. The standing-up mirror position is best with a full-length mirror that's on the wall alongside you. You lean forwards against the wall that's at right angles (look, it's really not as complex as it sounds), while he enters you from behind holding onto your waist, thus giving you both a fantastic view of his penis and your arse. If you're naked, you even get to see breasts, too.

---

then it's simply a great experience for both of you, as far as sensation goes. Alright, yes, you may sacrifice a little intimacy, but he can always look into your eyes later on, once the excitement's died down a little. All you do is get on all fours and stick your bum in the air. This is not dignified. But for your watching partner, it's deeply sexy. He enters you, holding on to your hips or waist, and can reach round to your breasts and clitoris. His penis will go in very deeply – so if you don't want to get pregnant, take steps to prevent it happening. The good news is it will hit your G-spot because the tight fit of entry from behind means all the vaginal nerves are touched. If you lie down with your bum still sticking up, the stimulation is even greater, and if you do it in front of a mirror, it's a great sight for both of you – it's about the only position in which you can both watch without cricking your necks.

cat

This is missionary with a much higher chance of female orgasm. If you have always orgasmed perfectly in missionary position, before returning to your knitting and bible study, then ignore this bit – but if you like the intimacy and closeness of him on top, but resent the fact that he gets to come like an express train, while you're left checking his bum for pimples, this is for you. The Coital Alignment Position is simple. He lies on top of you, penis inside you, as usual – then he inches up your body till he's as high as he can get, without bending his penis agonisingly. Then, instead of thrusting, he simply grinds in small circles. A lot of good sex relies on small circles, and this is just one example. This has the effect of stimulating your clitoris thoroughly, because he's moving right on top of it continuously – with normal missionary, he's just intermittently banging it, which is going to result in nothing more earth-shattering than painful bits.

Your orgasm relies on him grinding slowly – as soon as he gets overexcited, it's all over. So play with his balls, kiss him – anything to distract him from the desire to get all jiggy.

face to face

Now we're getting all *Kama Sutra* – this position looks exactly like a 16th-century wood-carving, and is elegantly symmetrical, compared to the kick-and-rush nature of most sexual couplings. All you have to do is sit facing him, on his lap. You wrap your legs over his hips and join your feet behind his bum to stay in place. He joins his feet so his legs provide a balancing platform for you. Once his penis is inside you, just rock, using his hands on the bed for balance if necessary – yours will be round him. It's the perfect position for kissing, he can reach your breasts, and your clitoris is stimulated by the pressure of his pubic bone. If you thrust too hard, admittedly, there is a chance of tipping over – but if you keep it slow and steady you can both build up to a thrilling climax. It also allows for a lot of neck-kissing, which is one of the most erogenous zones for both of you. Just be careful not to bang teeth when it gets passionate.

standing (backwards)

Standing-up sex can be a gateway to a world of disaster. If you aren't the right heights for it, you're basically a Chihuahua barking up a redwood when it comes wrong trees. However, there is a way round it – apart from high heels. If you're after a quickie, and lying or sitting down just isn't a pos-sibility in the dark alleyway you've found yourselves in, then you just turn round to face the wall, stand about two feet away from it, and stick your bottom out. He may have to bend down a little if your height discrepancy is big, but it's much easier for him than front-ways – if you try that, you have to get one leg up round his waist so he doesn't slip out, and stand on tiptoe, which might work for a trained ballerina but is something of a liga-ment-strain for the rest of us. This way, you have a wall to brace yourself against so he can thrust much harder, and better still, he can actually locate the right bit without too much trouble and knee-bending. Again, it's good for your G-spot, and allows him to reach your breasts – if you have time, before the policeman flashes his torch at the pair of you.

squatting

You thought doggy was undignified – this position makes it look like a Sothebys antiques auction in comparison. But it's worth it. Basically, he lies on his back, and you squat above him. Yes, squat, I'm afraid. Then he penetrates you, and you raise yourself up and down, using your hands on the bed – or his chest – for leverage. You mustn't lean forward, and you must balance on your feet, not kneel down. Yes, it will resemble constipation, but the idea is, you're at such a level of passion that neither of you will make that connec-tion. At least, not at the time at any rate. The beauty of this position is that it instantly provides full penile access to every area of your vaginal nerves. And as you plunge up and down – because that's what you need to do – with every thrust, they'll be stimulated beyond your wildest imaginings. It works – you just look, on some basic level, slightly stupid. But he probably won't care. And from the throes of your orgasm, neither will you. It allows him room to play with your breasts and clitoris – though he shouldn't do that while you're plunging or someone could have an eye out.

half off the bed

Some sexual positions require some sort of prop – even in cave times, they may have done things with bison bones that we don't even want to think about. But for this one, you only need the very basic prop of a bed.

You lie on your back, with your bum on the edge of the bed, and your legs on the floor. He stands up, and you wrap your legs round his waist, or at least hook your knees over his hips. He then holds your thighs, and thrusts into you, which allows for very deep penetration, and hard, passionate sex. The good part is, you hardly have to do anything, and he does all the work. He's pumping like a piston engine, you're lounging around – sounds good to me. It's a good G-spot position, too, because his penis will be rubbing against the front wall of your vagina, and again, it allows for lots of breast access. If you turn over and kneel up, his standing-thrust will give you a uniquely pleasing take on doggy position, too. The only thing required is some stamina on his part – he has to be the kind of man who doesn't go weak and jelly-legged due to exertion, or else you'll be collapsing in a feeble heap after two thrusts.

legs on shoulders

This is a great position all round, but only if you're slightly bendy. If you're not, you're looking at a locked back and a lot of tears and recriminations, so you may want to do some stretching exercises first, to ensure suppleness. Again, you lie on your back (there's a pattern beginning to emerge here ...) and he kneels between your legs. Then you raise your legs so your ankles are on his shoulders – unless you're a giantess, they'll fit perfectly, just make sure you don't kick him in the ear when he starts thrusting. He has full access to breasts and clitoris, and you can go as fast or as slowly as you like in this position. He can hold your bum to enable thrusting, or caress you. It's best if you don't attempt to do a whole lot, given that you're doubled up at the waist like a flick-knife, so your job is just to lie back and enjoy it. The angle again gives a great depth of penetration, and because he can see all your bits, it's a visual turn on for him. You can place your feet

> **TIP**
>
> You should never be embarrassed by the noises your body makes during sex, because men find them highly erotic – any squishy noises are part of the whole experience. You can get a similar effect from lubrication on your hands, so if you are using it, it doesn't hurt to rub them together first. Other noises – such as the charmingly named 'fanny fart' – are simply a result of having air forced into your vagina by his thrusting, and therefore nothing to be embarrassed about. In fact, it's his fault if anyone's.

against his chest too, to brace against thrusting, but if you do, remember to take your high heels off first, unless you want to end the session cutting up bits of bandage and apologising profusely …

her on top

It's old, it's familiar – but it works, without a doubt. The only negative when it comes to this position is the fact that you actually have to make some effort. This time, it's him lying back like Cleopatra on a burnished barge while you get down to the serious thrusting. But the advantage is, you get to control the pace – sometimes blokes go way too fast because they get all excited, bless them. For you, there's no danger of over-thrusting, it's just a matter of which position presses best on your clitoris. Try leaning forward slightly to grind your pubic bones together, or backwards if you want to expose it for rubbing. You can even rub it yourself if he isn't doing it to your satisfaction – or whip out a vibrator, and hold it between you, which is always a winner, whatever position you happen to be in. With you on top, you get great breast access, and he can fondle your bum. As you speed up, make sure you don't raise yourself too far before you plummet back, or you could miss altogether and do horrible things to his penis. Not desirable. Still, being on top allows you to rub and grind as much as you like – whereas a lot of positions mean you're in his hands as to speed and direction, this one enables you to control the pace to your precise specifications, which means you can also come when you like, roll off and fall asleep. It's only fair.

Now, with that repertoire of ten you could probably keep yourselves happy on a desert island for quite some time. But on a desert island you wouldn't have any props to enhance the experience with – so for a really good time, you'd ideally want a few ways of livening up the basic ten, with the odd twist here and there. So you may wish to investigate the following – and if you fall out and break your ankle it's no use suing me, I'm only telling you, not advising you …

advanced
chair

A simple chair can make all the difference to your sexual experience – but make sure it's a non-staining fabric. The ideal kind is a solid wooden kitchen chair that isn't going to tip over the moment you get giddy. He sits on it, and you sit on his lap, facing him. He's supported with his feet on the floor, and you are supported by him holding you up. You rock, holding onto the back of the chair (don't even think about trying this on a stool, it will end in disaster for sure) – he can't move much, but again, you get to control the pace, and grind your clitoris into him, which works nicely. You can try this with a rocking-chair as well, but be careful you don't both go flying during a particularly passionate session.

swing seat

This is a bizarre contraption rather like the kind of thing James Bond villains have hanging in their mountain lairs – 'Ha ha ha, Mr Bond, not so confident now?' – but having said that, it can offer a brand new take on the whole sex thing, and given that people have been doing it for several millennia now, that can't be bad. This swinging hammock with holes and straps hangs from the ceiling, and one partner sits in it while the other takes the opportunity to swing them around, thus gaining access to whichever orifice takes their fancy. It removes troublesome gravity from the situation, so it resembles having sex in space, but without the capsule food, or oxygen problem. Once again, 'dignified' isn't the word that springs to mind – but then, who cares when he has access to every single part of you, and can swing you around like some pornographic astronaut? The only drawback is, you'll have to tell your Mum it's a new Arne Jacobsen design when she comes to visit.

inversion

This position requires some gymnastic ability, but it's worth practising for the head-rush you get. You know how really, really stupid and/or reckless people believe that asphyxiation leads to a stronger orgasm? Well, this is the safe version where you don't get to die at the end of it. He sits on the edge of the bed, and you sit on his lap, facing him. Then you bend backwards, so your head is hanging down, and all the blood rushes to it. Make sure he's holding onto you tightly, though, or your giddy experience will revolve around the fact that he's just slammed your head into the parquet flooring. Don't attempt full sex in this position, you will go very dizzy indeed – but bending backwards as orgasm approaches should ensure an extra rush. Don't try him in the same position, however – you won't be able to hold him up and it will end up with him nursing a lump that won't be in his trousers.

actual swing

Some people swear by a real swing for their kicks. If you have sex on a swing – whilst swinging, obviously – the G-force rush as it flies up and down can intensify your orgasms. The main thing to be aware of is who's holding on, however – if both of you rely on the other, you'll be swinging straight into A&E without looking down. Ideally, he should hold the chains, while you straddle him, and hold onto him. You can't thrust much either, and unless you have a swing on your own private land – or in the bedroom – you do run a heavy risk of being arrested by an irate park keeper.

table

Far safer, the sturdy table is an ideal sexual prop. You can use it in the same manner as the bed, but you'll get a lot more friction out of it, as the hard surface will enable you to feel every thrust much more effectively. It will also enable your bum to ache much faster, being hard wood rather than yielding mattress – but it's surely a small price to pay for kitchen-based excitement. He should stand at the end, between your legs, and you should put your feet on two kitchen chairs – or one, and wrap the other one round his waist. If you don't support your feet, your back will start to hurt, and you'll be shunting up and down rubbing sore patches on your buttocks. Most importantly, be certain it's a well-made table. You don't want everything falling apart at the climactic moment in a shower of Swedish nuts and bolts.

car

To have sex in the car, there are a variety of options (but don't do what I did once, which was leave the engine running so we could have the radio on, only to get a flat battery and end up stranded in some car-park in the middle of nowhere at midnight …). To avoid some undignified *Rita, Sue & Bob Too* scenario with feet sticking out of the windows of your Morris Marina, you need to ensure your car is big enough. Then decide if you're going to succumb to passion in the front seats – which involves all sorts of bother with the gear stick, so unless it's an automatic, forget it – or climb into the back and go for it in relative comfort. The drawback of the back seat is that if you are interrupted, you have absolutely no excuse as to what you were doing. Nevertheless, it's far easier to get into a relatively comfortable position, so I recommend it. He should sit upright on the back seat, and you straddle him – but only if you're not being watched. If you're next to picnicking families in a car-park in midsummer, you need to lie down – him along the back of the seat, and you clinging onto him like a

---

TIP

If your relationship's gotten into a dismal rut, then sex expert Anne Hooper suggests making small changes at first that will alter the way you approach sex. So swapping the side of the bed you sleep on will automatically force a slightly different method into it, as will changing the hands you both use for hand jobs. If you wear a nightie and he wears PJs, go to bed naked, and if you always sleep naked, then wear something – ideally, something seductive. If you usually do it in the dark, switch the light on and vice versa … a change is as good as a rest, but it's also as good as a vastly improved shag.

baby marmoset, in the Scissors position. Don't even think about reclining the front seats. It absolutely does not work.

wheelbarrow

You do not need a wheelbarrow for this position, luckily. You do, however, need to cast your mind back to those playground wheelbarrow races, where some nine-year-old held your legs up and you staggered on your hands past the hopscotch markings to victory. This version, though, is even more exciting, if that were possible. For a unique sexual thrill, stand on your hands (naked, obviously) while he catches your legs, and places them on either side of his waist. Then he enters you, whilst holding you up. This gives him full and frank access to your entire bits; and you get the orgasmic head-rush from hanging upside down. You also get a locked spine, however, if you aren't damn careful, so make sure you don't attempt to hold the position for too long unless you are, in fact, a trained trapeze artiste. It does provide great access for G-spot stimulation, and if he's a bum-man, he gets a great view as well.

places to do it

The obvious and easy place to explore sexual positions is in bed. But while a comfy mattress provides an ideal base, you can have a lot more fun if you use the whole house (or even street, local park, shopping centre, supermarket aisle …) as inspiration for your sexual positioning. Some places are useless, naturally, by dint of the fact that they're too small, uncomfortable, or simply happen to be in front of your plate-glass windows that are overlooked by the neighbours (unless exhibitionism floats your boat, of course). There are, though, certain pieces of furniture or household fixtures and fittings that just lend themselves to wild sex. With the curtains drawn, obviously.

washing machine

The washing machine is a winner for sexual activity – not only can you give your dirty underwear a nice spin afterwards, but you get throbbing like no vibrator ever invented, so long as you make sure to balance on it as it approaches the spin cycle. The old-fashioned type, that judders and hums and jiggles as it cranks itself up to full power is best – that way, you get the sensation spreading from underneath your bum through your clitoris, when you sit on the top, and wrap your legs round his waist so he can enter you. It takes a little balance, and you must be certain it's not the kind of machine that's going to break and flood the kitchen in your excitement – but most vital, try and time your orgasm to happen before it moves onto 'final rinse' or you'll be left high and, er, dry.

sofa

If you want a little more excitement than that dull old bed, but you don't want to get nasty carpet burns, the sofa provides a great compromise. Best

---

TIP

At the beginning of your relationship you're up for doing it any-where – no surface goes untried. But after a while, the bedroom is the only place that gets to see any action apart from the domestic. You have to make an effort to meet in a different venue – such as the kitchen. A simple change from the bed to the kitchen table can result in an entire range of sensations that you don't get when you're lying on a soft mattress, and lends itself to a range of new positions. But if it ain't going to happen naturally, then make a con-scious decision.

position is either straddling him, or doggy, lengthways on the cushions. Or you can bend over the back while he enters you from behind, or lie in missionary position and fondle his bum. Be aware, though, that it's considered terribly bad form to watch TV out of the corner of your eye while he's struggling to give you an orgasm.

kitchen units

Kitchen units are useful because they're firmly built, and unlikely to collapse in the middle of your display of passion. You can perch on the edge while he stands between your legs, or lean on the counter while he enters you from behind. He can surprise you at the sink for a quickie – or more likely, you can surprise him – and what's more, there's a kettle within easy reach for the post-coital cup of tea.

shower

Having sex in water is largely overrated – it just ends up with everyone suffering from stinging eyes, and all the natural lubrication is washed away in a torrent of apricot shower-gel. However, there is a way to have sex in the shower, and get the whole 'soaping each other sensually' excitement going, without spitting a waterfall over each other at the same time. You need to sit, though. It all goes wrong when both of you try and stand up, and is also a recipe for cracked ribs when one person slips sideways on a loofah. So adopt the face-to face position, under the falling water, and rock gently – but use soap on each others' bits, because it stings like hell.

As for having sex in the bath, two words: don't bother. No orgasm is worth the amount of heaving around you're going to have to perform to find a position with a chance of working.

stairs

The stairs – or a flight of steps, as immortalised by Kim Basinger and Mickey Rourke in *9 1/2 Weeks* – are an interesting venue for sex. Being at different levels, they allow you to swivel your bodies around into new positions – if you're feeling wild you can hang upside down, or balance over him, as he sits down on them, with the higher stairs providing a handy shelf for holding on to. Of course, you may have a somewhat painful back, due to the ridges caused by lying along the flight – but the opportunities for contorting yourselves are impressive, and it certainly adds a *frisson* to basic missionary when there's the chance you'll start sliding downwards if you thrust too hard.

games

There are various sex games you can play – anything from Key Parties to Strip Chess – but the Dice Game is the best when it comes to positions.

You get two dice – for the first, write down a series of sexual positions. I suggest:

- missionary
- doggy
- spoons
- her on top
- standing up
- wheelbarrow

For the second, write down six venues – such as:

- kitchen table
- on the stairs
- on the washing machine
- in the car
- in bed
- on the sofa

Then take turns throwing both – and the rule, of course, is that you must do exactly what it tells you. Even if that's 'on the stairs, wheelbarrow'. Throw again when you've either managed it, or broken your ankle – whichever comes first.

3   orgasm

Orgasm is the holy grail of sex, the explosion that it all leads to, and the main cause of problems, at least as far as women are concerned. Because we're all so focused on coming, scoring the winning goal, waves crashing on the shore, wild horses galloping along the beach and every other cinematic image that was ever crassly used to suggest orgasmic union, the pressure to come – regularly and spectacularly – is enormous. The truth is, however, that most women vary when it comes to coming. At certain times of the month, generally mid-cycle, you may have wild, porn-star orgasms with the merest flicker of the clitoris – but if you're tired, stressed, or pre-menstrual you can be on a *chaise longue* with the entire England rugby team and a well-thumbed sex manual and still be feeling nothing more than a faint sore patch somewhere down below.

Female orgasm is a gentle flower, that needs to be unfurled slowly and kindly – of course, there will be times when you just want a violent quickie, and you may come dramatically from the sheer thrill of it all, but generally speaking, if he's giving it a couple of thrusts and then asking 'Are you close?' the whole thing will sputter out in damp-squib feelings of inadequacy.

It isn't just women who suffer from orgasmic performance anxiety, either – men, while toting their orgasmic equipment around a little more obviously, are still supposed to be able to come after a few manly strokes and all advice focuses on delaying, not speeding up, their orgasms. Nevertheless, sometimes men can suffer equally from 'why isn't it happening' syndrome – tiredness, stress and drunkenness affect men too, and his orgasm can be inhibited by any of these factors. (Of course, if you've recently said 'hahhaha, what's that pant-peanut?' upon viewing his penis, that may also explain his inability to truly let go …)

Still, the accepted wisdom is that if you rub your bits together, lick each others' bits or touch each others' bits for long enough, you will both, eventually, explode in a shower of spangles and gasping. And while that may well be the case, there are ways to ensure orgasm is more enjoyable, less long-winded and less pressurised for both of you.

orgasm for her

Orgasm for you, in a good 70% of cases, is down to having your clitoris stimulated. This is the bottom line, that whatever other pyrotechnics you may engage in, whatever superior brand of penis he's got, it won't make a darn bit of difference if he's ignoring your clitoris in favour of concentrating all his attempts on your vagina. While the vagina is, admittedly, great at responding, filled as it is (at least for the first 3 inches) with nerve endings, G-spots and what have you, the clitoris is a far more sophisticated little device. While the multi-tasking vagina is there basically to let sperm in, and babies out, the clitoris is the only human organ constructed solely for the pleasure of the owner. Really – there's no other reason for it than total enjoyment. If the vagina is the house, the clitoris is the wine bar next door, pumping out loud music, filled with laughing revellers having a great old time.

It doesn't just consist of the little pea-like bit you can see – it's like a baby penis, and stretches along under the skin of your labia for a few centimetres, which explains why it feels so great to have your inner labia fondled by his finger, on the way down to your vagina. The whole area is packed with nerves, too, so if he focuses on the clitoris and its immediate environs,

Many people, however intimate they've just been with their partner, avoid looking at each other when they come. It's such a deep and personal moment, it takes a lot of trust to share it. But watching your partner come is also very exciting and erotic – and can encourage your own orgasm. Tell him you'd like to look into his eyes, so he doesn't shut them and turn his head away, and you must be prepared to let him do the same. You will not look silly – it'll probably be the most erotic thing he's ever seen in his life.

he can't go far wrong. Actually he can – see 'hand jobs: pressing too hard,' for details – but the real mistake is dismissing the whole thing as just an unnecessary bit of skin, and going straight to vagina without passing 'Go'. Of course, it plays a part – but it's not the be-all and end-all to female orgasm.

orgasm during intercourse

Foreplay is vital for women's orgasm – if the rest of you isn't aroused, nine times out of ten, your bits won't be either. See 'Foreplay' for details of what to do. But once you're heading down the road to sensation, it takes a big problem to set you off course. One such problem is the fact that most sexual positions fail to stimulate the clitoris steadily – so he's bashing away, wondering why you're not beside yourself with excitement, when what he should be doing is stimulating your clitoris at the same time. Now, admittedly, this takes practice. Most men are simply not dextrous enough to manipulate a clitoris sensitively whilst keeping up a respectable level of thrusting. So you either need to get into a position that allows him full access to rub you without any sudden jerky moves – or else you can do it yourself.

positions

Best positions are Scissors – he can reach down between your legs and it's impossible to move too fast in this position anyway – or him kneeling, you on your back with your legs spread. That way he can see exactly what he's doing, and touch your clitoris without any sudden lurching moves that are going to spoil everything. You on top can also work, if he spreads his hand on his stomach and uses his thumb to press on your clitoris as you rock.

It's possible in doggy position, but as it lends itself to urgent thrusting, it's not ideal.

diy

Of course, you could simply opt to save him the bother altogether by masturbating yourself while he busies himself with the thrusting part. It may feel like he's getting off lightly (as it were) but look at it this way: you're getting touched the way you like best, and you aren't going to have to spend the whole time muttering 'harder', 'no, softer', 'bit to the left, please' when you're simply trying to concentrate on coming as effectively and enjoyably as possible.

There aren't many positions that don't lend themselves to a little self-starting, but missionary doesn't work too well, it has to be said. With everything else, if you can hold on one-handed, you can touch your own bits – then he simply has to match his hip movements with your hand movements, or vice versa.

The 30% of women who do come through vaginal intercourse are usually lucky enough to have clitorises that are closer to their vaginas, so the movements inside have a ripple effect on the clit itself. Which will not happen if it's situated miles away at the top of your labia, which is more common.

It seems obvious – but that never stopped anybody ignoring something. A simple but highly effective sex trick is simply to act like you're turned on. Presumably, you're already a little involved, or you wouldn't be there in the first place. But if you need a little extra, writhe around passionately, gasp when something feels good, and groan when it feels great. Talk to each other – saying 'you're so sexy' can elevate the experience from basic sex to really great sex, simply because it makes you feel your partner's focused entirely on you. It's not about faking – just appreciating what's there more effectively.

the g-spot

One way of coming vaginally (if it's something you're very keen to do of course) is to locate and utilise the elusive G-spot.

Some believe that the G-spot is merely a myth created by men (Dr Graftenberg to be precise) to enable them to slack when it comes to ensuring female orgasm. If he can lie back and say 'Listen darlin' I was going like a steam train and I didn't find no G-spot,' then the fact that you didn't have a vaginal orgasm is in no way his fault. It's certainly worth looking for, in the way that the remains of Alexandria are worth looking for – but even if you've devoted the time, paid your teams of diving experts, and mapped what you're looking for to the last co-ordinate, no one's going to be at all surprised if you return empty-handed.

Still, if you're determined to mount the expedition, if you'll forgive the pun, then the basic things we know about the G-spot are these.

Some women claim they have them – but only about one in five would swear to it. It is located about 4 inches up on the front inside wall of the vagina, and feels like a spongy little jelly tot to the touch. To reach it – in theory – he needs to point his fingers inside your vagina towards your bum, and cup your bits. Then he should extend one or two fingers upwards, with the tips now curved over and pointing forwards to your stomach. Look, no one said this was easy, alright? Then, with a fingertip, he must fossick about up there until he locates said spongy bit.

Now this is where it gets more difficult. Because if his fingers aren't long enough, he can poke around up there for days and it's not going to make a blind bit of difference. If they are, and he magically chances upon a spot that when touched, makes you come over all hot and flushed, then by George, he's got it. You'll know, trust me, should he find it.

If so, he should just move the tip of his finger around very gently in – you guessed it – small circles. It will intensify your orgasm if he does this while simultaneously touching your clitoris with the other hand, in the manner of a Swiss watch-maker winding two masterpieces at once.

There are certain sexual positions which stand a fair chance of stimulating the G-spot (if it exists) – most notably, doggy position, which allows his penis to rub your front vaginal wall (and my that sounds so sexy, too …)

Your ankles on his shoulders can also work well, if he's leaning forward so his penis is pushing in and out at the right angle to stimulate the spot.

Supposedly, the G-spot orgasm will drive you insane with crashing waves of sensation – but as so few women actually know when they've had one, it may actually amount to nothing more than a pleasant sneezing sensation. Only you will know. and if it doesn't work, at least the clitoris is ready and waiting as back-up.

the a-spot

You'd be forgiven for thinking that now they're just making the damned spots up. Hey, I think I'll come up with a few ... what about the P-spot halfway up the sphincter ... or the Z-spot, which sends you to sleep when pressed ... Still, we're nothing if not thorough, so we will accept that such a thing as the A-spot may actually exist, and go in search of it accordingly. Lou Paget, who knows about these things, says that the A-spot is another wellspring of pleasure, at least potentially, and to find it, you must go past the G-spot – no, I don't know how either, unless you've got fingers like Mr Tickle – until you locate a sensitive spot about an inch further up. When stimulated, apparently, it can be responsible for the most intense vaginal orgasms. Then again, if you manage to get that far up and distinguish the A-spot from every other bit of spongy flesh up there, you probably deserve the kind of orgasm that still leaves you speechless three days later.

As far as A-spot positions go, your big chance is to shove a cushion under your bum, and place your ankles on his shoulders – so your hips are as high as they can get, and the angle of penetration is very deep

---

TIP

Lou has in her bag of tricks a Crystal Wand – a long, translucent vibrator that bends slightly at the end. The great thing about it is the little bend at the tip – which means it has a far bigger chance of actually reaching the A-, or even the G-, spot than, say, just to take a random example, his penis. So either he or you can insert it, then rotate or jiggle it gently, until it makes contact with something that feels exciting. And if it doesn't, then hey, you can always use it to unblock the sink.

indeed. And even then – well, you'll be lucky. But give it a try, you never know, right?

the u-spot

No, really, it exists … honest. And the good news is, to find this one, you really don't need a fully trained Sherpa. U is simply short for urethra, and to find it just let his fingers travel a centimetre or so down from the clitoris. It's recommended that you empty your bladder before commencing the search, because otherwise, the slightest pressure could just have you desperate to rush for the toilet. Once you've homed in on the spot, which is right underneath the clitoris, all he has to do is stroke it lightly for those familiar old orgasmic sensations to rise up. This is a spot that comes into its own during oral sex (see below) but can be touched with his finger while he stimulates the clitoris at the same time. The position that works best here is the 'frog' – back to the old undignified squat – where you crouch over him. But this time, while squatting, you lean forward slightly, so his groin is rubbing up against your U-spot – ideally his penis will be jiggling your G-spot, and frankly, the whole thing is just one big spot-stimulation.

TIP

For U-spot stimulation, the 'frog' position is best. You should squat over him, balancing on your feet rather your knees, while he lies on his back, and rub up against the base of his penis. The U-spot is only a centimetre or so from the vagina, so this should allow it at least to make contact. You need to be in control here, because the urethra is every sensitive and too much pressure can be a direct ticket to a bout of cystitis, which is no fun whatsoever.

oral for her

This is where it gets good. Oral sex is still banned in certain states of America – presumably because they know that when it's done right, nobody bothers going in to work, and state economics grind to a standstill. As far as good-god-I-can't-breathe-or-see orgasms go, oral sex is your best hope by a mile. The best thing about it is, you don't actually have to do anything, unless you're attempting the 69 position, which is far too complex to give you a great orgasm with ease. Most of the time, though, you're only required to lie back, legs apart, and occasionally run a hand through his hair while he licks you to giddy heights of unimaginable pleasure. At least, that's the idea. Unfortunately, however great in bed they may be, a lot of blokes think that all they have to do to get you all breathless is to lick in the general area of your bits with all the finesse of a Great Dane at a water bowl. And while it's hard to make being given oral sex actively unpleasant, it's not as easy as it looks to ensure it results in orgasm.

the wrong way

The wrong way for him to give you oral sex is for him to sigh, murmur 'suppose I'd better,' and flick your labia apart as if he's finishing off some irritating filing. Then he should definitely not proceed with a short series of giant licks, administered fairly harshly, after which he will struggle upwards wiping his chin and say 'are you nearly there, then?'

Men have to understand that a woman's bits are a delicate thing, and they no more respond to violent rubbing and licking than would a kitten. Also, if you aren't feeling right mentally it's almost guaranteed you won't come though oral sex – because it's so intimate, if you're feeling remotely worried about the smell, taste, look, feel, or, er, sound of your most womanly

TIP

The nipple orgasm may or may not be a myth. But just in case it isn't, the way to get one is, apparently, for him to suck gently on your tongue and lips, then exert the same pressure on your nipples, for the same amount of time. He may need to do this several times, but whether or not you actually have an orgasm, it's certainly going to feel pretty good. As a compromise, unless you have stunningly sensitive nipples that orgasm at the flick of a switch, he can also touch your clit.

bits you'll never relax enough to breathe properly, let alone come. Just remind yourself that most men are hard-wired to find the whole package desperately attractive, and if he doesn't, either you haven't washed for a good couple of weeks, or he's starting to become strangely fascinated by men in leather caps and moustaches.

the right way

The right way is for him to kiss his way down your body, finally approaching your bits as though they are the best chocolate saved from the box just for him. Small noises of lust and appreciation work very well. He should kiss them all over, then very gently use his finger and thumb to slightly part your labia, which has the effect of exposing your clitoris more effectively, and allowing more of it to be stimulated.

Then, if he's simply opting for the basic stimulation method (see below for 'Advanced'), he should flicker his tongue across your clitoris, and down to your vagina a couple of times, before returning to your clit and making tiny circles around it with his tongue, in a steady, gentle rhythm. He shouldn't take his tongue away at any point, and he certainly shouldn't stop to pick pubic hairs out of his teeth, which just has the effect of making him look like a 17th-century king picking wren bones from his molars, and is hopelessly unsexy.

He must just keep going, and be led by your gasps – if you push at the back of his head, he should assume you want the pressure harder, and if you pull him by the ears, he can surmise that you want it softer. He can also slide a finger into your vagina as he goes, but some women find this distracting, so be sure to tell him if his finger-work is taking your concentration off what his tongue's doing.

If he's really co-ordinated, he can reach up and play with your nipples – for many women this drives them completely over the edge, but only if you can shake the mental image of him being stretched on a rack as he juggles with all your bits at once. Shut your eyes, and forget what it looks like is my advice. When you come, he should be guided by you – if your clitoris has suddenly gone deeply sensitive, he should move away, but not so suddenly that he's implying 'thank god that's over' – a few more little kisses in the general area should serve as reassurance.

advanced methods
the kivin method

Lou Paget has a method of oral sex that almost guarantees orgasm every time. 'David Beckham and Brad Pitt come and stand naked at the end of the bed …' (nah, just kidding). It's called the Kivin method – not the Kevin method, though you can call it that if you wish. And it's fairly simple for him to do.

There are three points he needs to focus on – the ones on either side of the clitoral hood (the little bit of skin that conceals the clitoris when it's not in use) and one on the perineum (the bit that joins your bum with your vagina). He needs to place one finger on the perineum, and move his tongue across the two points, while two fingers are held on either side to expose your clitoris.

The other difference between this and more conventional methods is that for the Kivin method, he isn't lying between your legs – instead, he's lying at right angles to your body, with his head pillowed on your thigh. This makes it less likely that he'll press too hard, and also means you can touch him more easily. In fact, it's a winner all round – and according to Lou, if he gets it right, you can have several orgasms in a row, or what's commonly known as a 'multiple orgasm'.

multiple orgasm

A multiple orgasm simply means having more than one orgasm in a single sex session, via whatever method happens to be available. It does not necessarily mean the biggest orgasm of your whole, entire life (see 'full body orgasm', Chapter 8, for details on that one).

TIP

For a higher chance of multiple orgasms, you need to practise on building up your PC muscle. If you spend five minutes a day for three weeks tightening and releasing your PC muscles – the ones that you stop a wee mid-flow with, or unscrew bottle caps with if you happen to be an exotic dancer in a Thai bar – this amount of practice will result in a spectacularly tightened muscle, which will result in more orgasmic sensations when he's inside you. It will also ensure you never wet yourself when you sneeze, though that's probably not a big worry for you yet.

To heighten your chances of getting more orgasmic, you'll need to tighten up your PC muscle, which is the muscle you can feel when you squeeze as if you're stopping a wee from emerging. To do this – also known as Kegel exercises – just locate and squeeze, in bouts of 5 minutes. Yes, alright, it's a little tedious, but no one can see you're doing it, and it tightens your vagina beautifully.

It means that you can grip his penis harder – which, in turn, means you get more friction. But more importantly, it means that when you start to come, you can use those muscles to squeeze and release several times, which will, theoretically at least, allow your orgasm to peak and dip several times, before it finishes.

If you can keep going for one after another, he should let you recover for a few minutes – at least one minute, at any rate – till the extreme sensitivity subsides a little from your clitoris, then he can use his tongue to stroke gently alongside it. Extreme gentleness is the best way to get more than one orgasm – fingers are a little rough after the first, so mouth is a much better bet.

his orgasm

His orgasm is basically a whole lot simpler to deal with. The fundamental equation is, rubbing long enough = orgasm. But there are ways of doing it that will, inevitably, result in better, quicker or slower, depending on which you prefer, orgasms for him.

during sex

Orgasming during sex is, for him, the main goal – and it is, shall we say, a whole lot easier for him to come this way than it is for you. He needs

TIP

To prolong his orgasm, and even extend it to multiple status, he also needs to work on his PC muscles. In his case, this gratifyingly involves watching him drape a washcloth over his penis and attempt to lever it up and down, for five minutes a day. Hilarious entertainment though this is – and you may want to construct some rope and pulley systems whereby he can winch toy cars up and down – if he gets really good, it also ensures that he will last longer when he's inside you.

simple friction against his penis, and as the vagina provides perfect friction all the way round, not to mention the warmth and wetness he's come to associate with orgasm, it's usually inevitable that he will come. If you'd like to slow down his headlong rush to ejaculate, though, there are certain positions that improve his chances of hanging on just that bit longer. Long enough for you to start enjoying yourself, at any rate.

Deep penetration positions where he gets to thrust hard and fast are obviously no good for delaying his orgasm. The best types are those that require him to go at your pace, and can accommodate occasional stops and starts.

You on top is ideal, as you can just sit there squeezing your PC muscles for a while, ensuring he still has a good time, but unless they're like a python's stomach muscles it's unlikely he'll come through this method alone. Then when you do allow him to move, you can raise yourself up slightly to stop him penetrating you with the whole shaft, because stimulation of just the tip is also unlikely to make him explode immediately. When it's time, you can move up and down suddenly, which is almost guaranteed to have a thoroughly orgasmic effect.

Another useful position is the face-to-face, as again, you're in control of the depth of penetration. If you want him to come sooner, just choose a position that allows for deep penetration, and whose pace is controlled by him – missionary or doggy, for example.

intensifying it
anal bits

To intensify his orgasm, there are various tricks you can master. And a disturbing familiarity with his prostate gland is just one of them. This little bean-shaped organ is situated towards the top of his anal passage. Lovely news so far, I agree. But if you aren't too squeamish about stuffing a well-lubricated finger up there, you can caress it as he thrusts, or even as you give him a blow job. Be gentle, he can be sensitive up there – but pressing lightly on it as he's about to come can noticeably increase the strength of his orgasm.

The perineum is a useful place to press, too, being rich in nerve endings, and close to said prostate – but do not press too hard, or it may well all go horribly wrong, and end in tears of agony rather than gasps of excitement. Just press it as you would a lift button – enough for it to light up, not enough for it to malfunction altogether.

Some men love the sensation of having their anus pressed while you're touching their penis or having sex – but best check first, in case he's got some deep-seated paranoia about it, and the merest brush of finger on anus results in a flaccid willy and an embarrassed man.

balls

Balls are a tragically neglected area, but they are highly sensitive little organs, and should be treated with respect and affection. If you stroke his balls while you stimulate his shaft, it can make his orgasm the greatest, most contented spontaneous explosion of feeling since England won the World Cup. They have a little ridge running up the middle, which responds very well when stroked or licked. If you can fit one or both into your mouth (though obviously not while you're having sex), this feels fantastic for him, and will almost certainly result in spectacular orgasm if you're stimulating his penis at the same time. You can even hum on them – you will feel utterly stupid, obviously, but it will have the same effect as a small vibrator, which feels great for him. Don't hum 'Colonel Bogey' though (otherwise known as 'Hitler Has Only Got One Ball').

The only thing you have to remember with his balls, though, is Tread Carefully. It doesn't matter what amazing things you're doing to the rest of him if you're being too rough with them – he will register only pain. So never bite, chew, flick, tap or squeeze them. Other than that, you're free to fondle, caress, lick, suck, stroke and blow on them with abandon, though don't be surprised when they suddenly shrink to half the size and rise upwards – it simply means he's about to come.

the basic blow job

It really isn't difficult to give a blow job – at worst, it can be mildly uncomfortable – for you, not him. It's only uncomfortable for him if you clamp your teeth together while you're doing it.

All you have to do is put his penis in your mouth, and lick and suck. But if you're hoping he'll enjoy a great orgasm at the end of it, you may require a little more in the way of technique.

The best position for giving a blow job is either crouched between his legs, him sitting – a little porn, I know, but we're talking about what's most

If you have long hair, it's very sensual for him if you wrap strands of it round his penis and stroke it up and down over the head – you can even give him a hand job with your own hair wrapped round him, for friction. The smell and texture of your hair can be a real turn-on for him – some men even have a hair fetish – so don't ignore it as a sexual tool. If you haven't got long hair, you can achieve a similar effect with a silk scarf. And it's not as difficult to wash when he comes all over it, either.

comfortable for you here – or lying, as he does in the Kivin method, at right angles to his body, with your head pillowed on his thigh, as he lies on his back. Never attempt to give him a blow job whilst lying between his legs, you'll get the most appalling crick in your neck halfway through, if not before.

Begin by circling your tongue on the tip of his penis, while placing your hand around the base. This is a highly useful move, as you can use this to elongate the length of your mouth – you're never going to get six inches in without gagging, so if three inches are being attended to by hand, it's much more manageable for your mouth, and he knows no different. Deep throating is a myth – and as the average man's penis measures 5¾ inches and the average woman's mouth is 3 inches, it's just as well. Now, slide your mouth over the shaft, and close your lips over it, tucking your teeth firmly away. Move up and down, angling your head so you're hitting the inside of your cheek rather than your throat with the tip. Suck lightly, but not so hard it makes your cheeks ache. Occasionally flicker your tongue along the sensitive ridge that runs along the front of his penis, and pay a little attention to the frenulum with the very tip of your tongue. As he gets more des-

TIP

For a very dirty and porn-friendly version of sex (ideal for, say, when you've got your period) you can give him a tit job. There may be a man out there who doesn't like this, but he's probably listening to a Judy Garland album right now. So he puts his penis between your breasts, you squeeze them together with your upper arms – or if you have small breasts, your hands – and he thrusts away. You can use body oil or KY to make it smoother – and of course, you may be able to bend your neck forward so you can lick the tip as he thrusts upwards. There's every chance he'll want to come on your face – or you can be a really kind porn-star and take him in your mouth, the choice is all yours.

perately eager, he will thrust and leap like a spawning salmon in a bid to get further into your mouth. Your hand will stop this happening, so make sure you're moving it in rhythm with your mouth, and failing that, a gentle flex of the jaw can help.

The faster you go the better as he approaches orgasm, but don't adopt such a breakneck pace you're going to collapse exhausted thirty seconds before the finishing line. Keep up a regular, steady beat, and move your hand faster rather than your neck, while increasing your sucking pressure. And he will, almost certainly, come.

You can elaborate on this blow job, but it doesn't need much embellishment, so if you feel like moving up and down flicking your tongue up and down the main vein, or twisting your head slightly as you reach the tip, to give him extra sensations, go right ahead – but if you don't, he still won't complain.

spit or swallow?

The eternal question – it's entirely up to you. But if you are going to swallow – which is nicer for him, even if it's not for you – let it hit the back of your throat, collect it all there while he finishes, then swallow it down in one like a teaspoon of jelly. Otherwise, you'll be wondering whether you really should hate the taste quite that much, and imagining all the little baby sperms swimming excitedly down your gullet looking in vain for something to fertilise.

If you do it this way, trust me, you won't feel a thing. If you'd rather spit, you're in good company – about 60% of women are with you on that one.

multiple for men

Men can feasibly have multiple orgasms – but they generally can't ejaculate more than once so their ability to have multiples is reliant on their control of our old friend the PC muscle. In men, this is the muscle that's working when their penis twitches involuntarily (just say 'Kylie' to him if you need a demonstration of this in action). If he squeezes it just as he's about to come, once it's strong enough it can actually prevent him ejaculating – he'll experience all the rush of an orgasm without the end result – and if he has sex again shortly afterwards, he can experience prolonged orgasmic feelings. In theory, he can keep going, squeezing, and starting again. So book in a month or two off work if you're planning on teaching him the method.

4 spicing it up

In the first six months of a relationship, as well as labouring under the belief that you both agree on your musical tastes and could never have a row, you're almost certainly having sex as though hell-bent on repopulating the planet in the nuclear aftermath. This is for various reasons – like you haven't yet noticed his habit of turning his pants inside out to wear them for two days, and he hasn't chanced upon your Phil Collins collection – but more importantly you're both flooded with PEA, the Love Hormone, which tells you that you must make love 24/7 because you two are the only people on the planet who have ever understood the point of sex. This subsides after a while, because if it didn't, you'd never get any work done due to your compulsion to lick each other's crevices while other people are hunched over their desks earning money.

The trouble is, once it's worn off, you still need to like the idea of having sex. Many couples attempt all kinds of drastic things to make sure the spark doesn't flicker and die, from affairs to plastic surgery to counselling – but the good news is, there are several much easier ways of spicing up your jaded sex life without having to pay thousands of pounds in court costs and therapists' fees.

The problems usually begin when real life has intruded good and proper – say, by way of children, or work, or general exhaustion – and it's perfectly common to find your partner somewhat less devastating than you did at first, once you're used to their snoring, duvet-stealing ways. But as long as you still fundamentally like each other, and aren't creased with loathing over the way the other eats soup, or rustles the newspaper, then it's worth pursuing a more exciting sex life, rather than giving up and running away with somebody else, with whom you'll be flooded with PEA for six months, only to realise that they steal the duvet too.

spontaneity

Being spontaneous takes planning, right? It's all very well sex manuals telling you to surprise him by opening the door naked, say – but first you have to have a shower, shave your legs, make sure it really is him at the door, check no neighbours are going past, and assume that he isn't too knackered to appreciate your little display. Planning is a good idea in most cases – besides, thinking about it in advance can succeed in turning you on in advance, too.

Obviously, you don't have to pre-arrange the whole thing like a military campaign, but it helps to have an idea of the mood, or what you're aiming for – it's no good presenting him with a sudden two-hour massage session if what he really wants is to watch the football. If you want to be

---

TIP

Men love to be surprised – so if the mood takes, you, grab him when he's got nothing more sexual on his mind than cooking pasta (though in certain 'specialist' shops I believe you can buy penis-shaped pasta …), undo his trousers, and give him a blow job. However, do not do this a) if you're beside an uncurtained window, b) if he's holding a pan of boiling water, it'll land on your head for sure, or c) if he's in a meeting at work. Other than that, go, girlfriend.

truly spontaneous, however, most men won't complain if you offer them a blow job at any time of the day or night.

On the whole, though, it pays to plan your sudden sexual moments to the point that you know you're both going to appreciate them.

Of course, this doesn't stop you sidling up behind him and kissing his neck – we're talking about spontaneity that demands an immediate response. If he 'spontaneously' books you into a hotel, that's great – but not if you'd arranged to go to a party with your best mate the same night. So small, unexpected gestures are perfect, but enormous, complicated unexpected ones are not quite so good.

planning sex

Planned sex sounds about as sexy as an obstetrics clinic. Passion isn't the first word that springs to mind, it's true, when you think of pre-arranging your sexual moments – but if you leave it to chance, chance can stretch

TIP

Send him a series of sexy text messages throughout the day, to keep him all worked up. Obviously, it helps if he knows they're from you – otherwise he might not mention them and then you'll think he's having an affair … god, it's way too confusing. But assuming he does know, just send him a few straight-to-the-point little thoughts like 'want 2 fck?' or 'u make me horny' or, for the shyer young lady, a simple, 'can't w8 2 c u'. If he comes home and says 'what were all those nonsense messages about?' assume he doesn't understand text language, and show him what you meant instead.

on for a good couple of months, unfortunately. By agreeing that you'll devote an evening to each other, you set up a certain expectation – but not so much so that you feel like the *Countdown* clock is hanging over your heads, ready to kick into action the moment the bottle of wine's opened. Because you don't have to grimly agree to sex – you're just giving yourselves the opportunity to have sex should you want to. Normally, you stagger to bed so tired you're lucky if you can pick up a book, let alone each other's genitals. This way, you're focused on what else you might do in bed. You can make it like a date; text him to arrange to meet him in the bedroom, and chill some wine (unless it's red, in which case it'll taste disgusting). Then you can kick off proceedings by giving him a massage, and with luck, he'll offer one in return.

After that, it doesn't take a scientist to figure out what goes where.

changing the routine

One of the most obvious problems behind sexual boredom is the fact that sex quickly becomes part of the same old routine. For a start, most couples nearly always have sex in the bedroom – which, with its peeling posters and overflowing laundry basket, is rarely the most desirable place to do it. And if you're in the same old familiar place every night, it's hardly surprising if you're having the same old familiar sex as well. It's ridiculously easy to slip into a series of moves more well-worn than an end-of-pier comedy routine – quick snog, breast fondle, a play with each others' bits and straight onto intercourse, strictly in the missionary position, followed by sleep. It's a rare couple that are still bending themselves into paperclip shapes in a bid for sexual union after the first few months – after all, why bother, when simply thinking 'I'll lie back and let him do the work' is so successful? Well, it's successful in that you'll orgasm because he knows exactly what to do, but it's not so good in the sense that you'll be so bored, half the time you won't want to bother in the first place.

The slightest changes can have a major effect on your sexual routine, because we appear to be programmed to respond to change by instigating more change. That's why middle-aged men don't just run away with their secretaries, they run away with their secretaries, and get a haircut that's too young for them, and buy a motorbike they can't afford, all at the same time.

So the idea is that if you change the environment you're having sex in, your sexual routine will get a handy shake-up too. This is certainly the case if you've decided to alter the venue to a lay-by on the M6. But as spicing it up goes, that may be pushing things a little too far. Ideally, you'll get rid of the kids/dog/friends for a night, and head straight for the nearest posh hotel, the best you can afford. There's absolutely no point in this whatsoever if your objective is to save money – because there's nothing less sexy than a miserable 2-star B&B, with fire regulations on the door and nylon bedspreads on the twin beds. You may as well stay at home and be uncomfortable for free.

But if you pool your resources, and can afford something half-decent with a nice shiny marble bathroom and a big bed, then you're already halfway there.

Just one night should be enough to revitalise things – but make sure you order room service, or midnight will strike and you'll still be waiting in the restaurant for your coffee. Oh, and get something delicate, there's no point stuffing yourselves on a gargantuan feast, and then falling asleep.

If you really can't afford a hotel, then do something different in the house – move the furniture around, buy some new bed linen, paint the walls a vibrant shade of pink – anything that improves the sex-quotient of your bedroom. Hell, you could even consider not letting the dog sleep on the end of your bed – it's all very cosy, but it's also slightly off-putting when Sadie the spaniel is gazing at you in innocent horror as you attempt to have a good time.

clothing

Along with changing the environment, you may wish to think about changing what you wear to the boudoir. That knackered old Mickey Mouse T-shirt you've been sleeping in for years may be cosy, but it ain't screaming 'Marilyn Monroe', is it? Now, I don't care how much of a card-carrying feminist you are, I'm one too, but that doesn't mean you have to dress like something out of *Eastenders*. Men are highly visual creatures, configured to respond instantly to an attractive sight – and you in decent lingerie comes somewhere near 'England score the winning goal' on his mental list of attractive sights. You may prefer the sensible white bra and pants combo,

---

TIP

Showering can be as dull and functional as teeth-cleaning. But it doesn't have to be. Next time he's singing 'Just One Cornetto' in the shower, jump in there – naked, dummy – and give him a full and thorough washing. Remember, though, if you do intend to move on to full sex, don't attempt it standing up – it'll all end in disaster. Just use your skills with the soap to make sure he's clean in every nook and cranny. Ideally, you'll use unscented shower gel – otherwise it can all get horribly stingy in his (and your) most intimate areas.

TIP

Don't leave sex till the evenings – you're both knackered. Studies show that afternoons are the best time to have sex, because that's when your hormones are at a peak. So what better way to liven up the day than to take an extended lunch hour and lure him home from work? You can always invent an urgent dental appointment. For both of you. A lunchtime quickie makes life so much more exciting than a weary roll just before sleep overtakes you – and you'll both go back to work feeling great. If you make it back, that is.

---

but rest assured, nine men out of ten prefer skimpy, black, lacy stuff, given the choice. And the tenth is just temporarily lost in some virgin-deflowering fantasy.

You don't have to spend fortunes on nice underwear – it's not going to be on that long. But you need a bra (avoid heavily padded cups, it's only disappointing for everyone when it comes off), a G-string (unless you have a mammoth-sized bottom, in which case French knickers are a good bet), a suspender belt (yes, I know, fiddly, time-consuming, pointless, but will drive him wild) and stockings. All men like stockings, particularly black ones. Don't think you'll meet him halfway and wear pop socks, incidentally – pop socks are the death of sex. You can also add high heels, and don't complain you'll look like a hooker – that's the point. It isn't giving in to the forces of sexist evil, it's just giving him a good time, and it's not as if he's really paying you. Chance'd be a fine thing. Dressing up shows you care about his enjoyment, and more importantly, that you still view yourself as a sexual being, which is a turn-on for you and him. Trudging to bed in frayed pants that say 'Monday' on the front (particularly when it's Thursday) and one of his

T-shirts does not suggest that you see yourself as anything other than a person who happens to sleep in the same bed as him.

Of course, he must return the favour by ensuring that he doesn't wear comedy boxer shorts from six Christmases ago ('hey, Father Christmas weeing! Thanks, Uncle Brian!') and that his underwear is clean, attractive and in no way bears a resemblance to something a male lap-dancer might wear. Boxers or trunks are harmless, wet-look posing pouches are not.

It goes without saying – almost – that hygiene should be of impeccable standards for both of you. But somehow I suspect he may need reminding slightly more often than you do.

stripping

Right, now forget you ever were a feminist for a moment, and consider making your partner dizzy with gratitude – by learning how to strip.

TIP

Men are visual creatures, we all know that, so what better visual thrill than you in underwear, or even naked? And to make it more exciting than the 'you in underwear' he gets to see every single night when you're chucking clothes on the bed, make it a surprise. Tell him you're 'just nipping upstairs to get something' while he's comatose in front of the TV … then reappear five minutes later in your best and sexiest lingerie and high heels. Naturally, he will understand your intentions immediately. Unless football's on, in which case he might murmur 'are you hot or something?' without taking his eyes off Beckham.

Wrenching off your clothes at the end of the day and shouting 'right, I'm off for a shower,' as he briefly glances up from the paper is not stripping.

Seductively removing each and every garment whilst gyrating to a suitably sultry tune and taking his breath away in the process, however, is.

Helen Jackson, an ex-stripper, runs classes, and has boiled the Perfect Strip down to a series of winning moves. With her expertise behind you, you won't feel stupid, clumsy or embarrassed, you will simply feel like a goddess luring him to your temple. Or at least, you'll feel quite sexy, and that can only be a good thing, right?

Wear a long dress that's easy to undo – no stripper ever looked good getting out of a polo neck and jeans. Under it, you need the full lingerie experience, plus elbow-length gloves and high heels to accessorise.

Choose your music – something with a good beat, but not too fast. Begin by standing with your feet together, sticking your bum out – think Bunny Girl.

TIP

A simple but effective tip – always dim the lights, or switch lamps on, when you're in the mood. There's nothing more passion-killing that a great big 100-watt bulb beaming down on you, highlighting every lump and bump and making the pair of you look like plucked turkeys ready for Christmas dinner. It might make you hungry, but it certainly won't make you horny. A couple of lamps in the corners should cast the sort of flattering glow that makes you look like a honey-skinned beauty, and create enough shadow to make the room look vaguely sensual rather than like an operating theatre.

When you're performing your striptease – or simply seducing him – it's vital that you show yourself off to the best advantage. So wear a high-cut G-string or knickers (high cut up the legs, that is, not the bum) to elongate your pins and make you feel tall and slim. Don't believe that stuff about hip-huggers 'giving you shape,' most men would infinitely rather look at you wearing pants that are held together by dental floss than admire the 'shape' created by large lycra knickers. Bridget Jones did not know what she was doing when it came to seduction – you, however, do, and all you have to remember is, the skimpier the better.

Now place your hands in the small of your back, so you're pushing out your breasts and bum simultaneously.

Dance for him for a little while (NB playing air guitar does not count and ruins the atmosphere). Keep eye contact – and don't laugh for god's sake. In fact, to avoid untimely giggling you may want to have a glass or two of champagne to get in the mood before you begin.

Make him believe you're about to remove a garment – and then take your hand away again … Start with your gloves. Pull each finger out, one at a time, taking four steps between each pull – then whisk the whole glove off and throw it to him to catch. He isn't allowed to touch you – so keep coming close then backing off. Unzip your dress and let it fall off your shoulders, pull it back up, turn round away from him and then let it drop to the floor.

Kick it aside, drop your bra straps, pull them back up … you get the picture. Every time you take something off, turn away, then turn back with your hands covering your body.

Flash your breasts at him and then cover them again … and wear high-cut knickers, because they make your legs look extra- long. You may wish to leave your shoes and stockings on – if not, make sure you wear hold-ups, and slowly roll them down. Suspenders are a stripper's nightmare.

Finally, when you're naked, keep your arms by your sides, pushing your cleavage together, jut one hip out … and after that, it's open season.

Of course, he could return the favour by stripping for you. And indeed, if you like that sort of thing, go ahead. But to many minds, the sight of a grown man gyrating to 'you can leave your hat on' whilst sliding his zip up and down, is just plain old daft, unless he's being paid to do it by a hen party. So perhaps leave the stripping to them as knows what they're doing, i.e. you.

danger

There is a pretty foolproof way of spicing up your sex life – which is, risking your life. Scientific studies have proven that the closer you come to danger, the more sexually aroused you are directly afterwards. So you per-

---

TIP

Call him at work and suggest he joins you for a 'quick lunch'. Say you've got something you want to ask him – though you may want to add that it's not 'can we have a baby,' 'can we move in together' or 'let's get married' – delete as appropriate. When you meet – whether that's at home or in a restaurant – say 'about what I wanted to ask you … fancy a fuck?' and lead him to the nearest bed/toilet cubicle/backseat of car. This is when quickies really come into their own.

> ## TIP
>
> Putting your leg up on a chair – or his lap – is a highly seductive move, as utilised by pole-dancers the world over, because it makes your legs look longer by tautening your thigh muscle, shrinks your bum, and makes you bend forward to show off cleavage. If you wear a long skirt with a split in it, which you can contrive to have fall open at the crucial moment, so much the better. And if you're not wearing anything, my god. Just don't expect him to be able to breathe for a good hour afterwards. If you're wearing high heels, though, a piece of advice – watch where you place your stiletto.

form a bungee jump, and seconds afterwards, you're ready to shag for Britain, in a desperate bid to procreate before you die – adrenalin is belting round your bloodstream, you're flooded with the joy of living, and the first thing you want to do is share your seed, or eggs, with the nearest person. Well, unless you're doing your jump for charity and emerge from your helmet to find that a beaming Jimmy Tarbuck is the nearest person you do, at any rate. So if you and your partner share a scary experience that gets your hearts pumping and your hormones racing, then you're much more likely to cling passionately together afterwards than you are if you've shared nothing but a boil-in-the-bag curry and a beer.

Obviously, major lifetime scary experiences aren't that useful for your sex life – canoeing down the rapids of Lake Victoria might be fantastic, but it's not the kind of thing you can do when you fancy a midweek shag. A good horror film (try *The Others* on DVD, I nearly cried with fright) or an exciting sports event – the proviso being that you both have to genuinely find it exciting – may well have a positive effect on your libidos, and revitalise your emotional responses. And if not, hey, you'll have something to talk about at the office tomorrow, even if it's not your sex life.

If horror movies don't float your boat, and *Coronation Street* just isn't doing it for you sexually, then consider having risky sex. Not the kind you have with a Brazilian transvestite named Venus and a shared syringe full of heroin; the kind where you could get caught. That's 'could', though, not 'probably will,' you'll note. So doing it in the back of a hired limo with a sliding screen is, for instance, better than doing it in the back of a hired mini-cab with a greasily fascinated driver. And doing it in deserted woodland is better than doing it in the grounds of a crowded National Trust property on a Sunday afternoon. The merest suggestion of 'someone could, potentially, come past and spot us …' is enough to add a *frisson* of extra excitement to your jaded sex lives. But don't let that *frisson* develop into a policeman and his three giggling sidekicks, will you?

Good places include deserted car-parks (without CCTV), beaches,

---

TIP

If talking dirty is a little embarrassing – and you live on your own together – get some sex fridge magnets. They enable you to spell out the filthiest comments – and even poems – imaginable, without ever actually having to voice your dirty sentiments. You can construct entire porn short stories on the fridge … but don't do what a friend of a friend did. Feeling frisky, he composed several thoroughly X-rated odes to his girlfriend's intimate loveliness and left it there for her to find next day. Forgetting, of course, that the cleaner was due at 9:00am. Who took it personally and promptly resigned … oh well, can't win 'em all.

other peoples' bathrooms at parties, and nightclub toilets at that stage of the evening when several people crowding into one cubicle is far from uncommon.

being sexy
underwear: lack of …

Being sexy is about more than simply leering 'alright sailor, what about it?', although there are certain situations where that can be a good start. But in a long-term relationship it requires a little more effort. Going out without knickers on is a good start, but remember to mention to him that you – oops! – forgot your underwear. Otherwise you'll just spend the night wriggling uncomfortably and he'll wonder why you appear so distracted. It helps if you wear a skirt that's short enough to be suggestive but long enough to stop you getting arrested for indecent exposure. He could go out without underwear too, but should he get an erection at an unfortunate moment, he's doomed, and will have to spend the remainder of his evening out with coats piled in his lap.

mirrors

If that seems a little too exposed, investigate the erotic potential of mirrors. Not on the ceiling, unless you suffer Bond-esque delusions – but a mirror positioned so you can see yourselves cavorting on the bed doubles your erotic fun. Anyone with the slightest hint of narcissism can get off on looking at themselves having abandoned sex, and if you don't think you're so hot, you can get a whole new view of your partner – when else do you get to see their arse thrusting into you? Oh, of course, the gang-bang video you made last New Year … but apart from that?

food

Eating food off each other is a perfect way to spice up your sex life – if you can rid yourself of the spectre of Alan Partridge smeared in chocolate, that is. There are, of course, certain foods that lend themselves to sexual shenanigans. Hot food doesn't generally come into this category – no one ever ate stew off each other convincingly. You might get away with melted chocolate – but see Alan Partridge, above, for reasons not to bother.

The ideal eating-off-people food is fruit, being, as it is, clean, sweet, and easy to eat in one bite. Alright, yes, it's a bit of a cliché, but if it didn't work, it wouldn't have become a cliché, think of that. Fruits you desperately need to stock up on for your night of – and I'm not going to sink so low as to say 'fruity passion' – love include strawberries, grapes, melon (in handy bite-sized chunks) raspberries, and, of course, bananas. The banana is for obvious reasons (no, not to compare his willy against …), but if you are going to insert it into yourself, try not to let it break off before he eats it out of you.

Pineapple rings are also nice to balance on his penis, though if they

---

TIP

Go supermarket shopping and fill a basket – or if you're feeling really frisky, a whole trolley – with foods you can eat off each other, or out of each other (banana-filled nostril anybody?). Suggestions include fruits such as strawberries, bananas and grapes, chocolate, honey, even licorice bootlaces to tie in bows round his willy if you so desire, and popping Space Dust, which is great for kissing, but painful for oral sex. You can also add ice cream, champagne, chocolate liqueur, puddings in your favourite flavour … just don't eat so much that you're too full to move. That's kind of not the point.

Food and sex is ideal for those who aren't too uptight about mess. If you are, you may as well forget it, because you'll never enjoy it – you're way too worried as regards sticky substances left on sheets for it to be worthwhile. Otherwise, you can just make sure you've got old sheets on the bed, and stick them in the washer afterwards. Do not, however, think you'll leave on the new Calvin Klein duvet cover and 'just be careful'– it'll be carnage, and the chocolate stains will never come out, so be warned.

actually fit over it, you're in trouble, size-wise. And be careful you don't get so absorbed in eating it you ignore the whole point of the exercise.

You can also involve liquids in your world of edible pleasure – champagne can be poured over each other and licked off, and it has the added bonus of smelling and tasting fantastic as well as getting you drunk and enabling your inhibitions to disappear entirely. You may think you shouldn't be inhibited with a long-term partner, but the more of a domestic life you lead, the harder it can be to let go of all your mental lists about taking the rubbish out and paying the milkman, and actually immerse yourself in simply being sexual. So yes, alcohol can help. But you didn't hear that from me, obviously.

If you are using champagne, be aware that the bubbles can sting like hell on your most personal bits – it's OK for him, as long as you don't pour it in the top, owwwwwww! The best way is to fill your mouth with liquid, close your lips over the top of his penis, and swoosh it around, before swallowing and commencing a blow job. God, he'll be your slave – at least for five minutes.

> **TIP**
>
> According to a scientific study, women are turned on by the smells of cucumber and licorice, and for men, pumpkin pie is a sensory excitement beyond measure. Don't even begin to ask me why, but the smells honestly send more blood to the genitals, thus sensitising them further. So try burning a cucumber-scented candle, or using Demeter cucumber perfume on your wrists, for a sensual charge. And it's surely possible to find something pumpkin-pie scented without having to cook the damn thing yourself.

He can do the same for you, licking it – quickly – out of your labia before it starts to sting. Or if that's too hardcore, off your breasts.

Tea and coffee are ideal blow job material – forget all that nonsense about ice cubes and chillies, just take a mouthful of hot (not boiling) liquid and repeat the champagne-swoosh manoeuvre.

Anything you ever read about or saw in a Madonna film, involving hot wax – forget that as well. It just hurts.

Honey is a great food for licking off each other – it's tasty, sterile, and apart from the ruined fixtures and fittings, it's convenient, particularly now you can buy it in squeezy bottles. But don't pour it on one another's hairy bits, it's a little too unpleasant to get out of the roots. As for peanut butter, forget it – that's just weird. Yoghurt is like being in bed with some wholefood-eating hippie (plus it smells funny), ice cream is too damn cold (though you can alternate a mouthful of ice cream and a mouthful of hot tea on the nipples/genitalia for a reasonably exciting effect), and cream has the same smell-problem as yoghurt. So don't bother stocking them in your erotic larder.

Vegetables must, of course, get a certain look-in. But only in the sense that if you want to do each other with carrots, that's entirely your business. Vegetables are not fundamentally sexual objects, but if you can find ways to press an aubergine – or, god forbid, a marrow – into service, then you go right ahead and do that. But make sure it's damn clean first – or possibly even peeled. But not diced, of course.

quickies

If you have hours at a time to devote to vegetable-based sex, that's just dandy and I'm happy for ya. But one reason most couples let sex slide to the bottom of the 'to do' list, right under 'buy new sink plunger' and 'get dog de-fleaed, is because they just don't have time at all. We have this belief that sex should be a fifteen-course banquet, lit with candles and surrounded by string quartets, and anything less seems like cheating. Well it's not. An orgasm is an orgasm, whether you arrived there after a five-hour coach

---

TIP

It sounds obvious, but it isn't – if you're going to tease him, or he's going to tease you, you really should follow through. Whispering 'when we get home I'm going to give you the best blow job you've ever had,' then bottling out and falling asleep is just mean. And if he promises a three-act massage, sighing 'yeah, but I wasn't tired when I said it,' it's far worse than welching on any other kind of bet – particularly if you're offering it as a bargaining tool. To avoid this, certain sex shops offer 'gift vouchers' for sexual services, whereby you fill one in, give it to him, and it has to be cashed shortly after being produced. It's only fair.

> ### TIP
>
> If sex simply isn't happening, because you're both too busy, and you can't even coordinate your diaries to ensure you're both in the same place at the same time, then you need to make a plan to have sex once a month. Once a month hardly sounds worth bothering with, but it's better than none a month – and quality in this situation is far more vital than quantity. Use it or lose it is also a truism when it comes to sex drive – so if you commit to at least one session a month it keeps you ticking over.

tour, or by supersonic jet, so it's a shame that quickies are so underrated. Women always think that quickies exist simply for the pleasure of men, that all they involve is her hitching her skirt up and him going 'uh-uh-uh-thanks, love,' but they're wrong. Quickies can be equally appealing to both sexes, because there's something deeply erotic about ignoring foreplay convention and heading straight for a good hard shag. You don't have to take your clothes off, as Jermaine Jackson once famously sang, to have a good time, oh no … I don't think that's quite what he meant, but still, leaving things on just adds to the urgency and excitement. The best quickie is unexpected – when he's just got in from work, say, pin him against the wall and relieve him of his trousers, then let him take you from behind. Or after a dinner party, sweep the empties to one side and do it on the kitchen table. You can even sneak round the back of a nightclub and do it under the fire escape, but you may well be interrupted by various drug dealers and their sniggering clientele, so go easy. A great time for a quickie is in your lunch hour – if you have time to sneak back home. Or if you're lucky enough to be having sex with a colleague, try the stationery cupboard at work.

Quickies are a great way of showing each other that you still want each other and desire each other passionately – and even if you don't, the good news is, you can invoke those feelings by going along with the idea, and seeing what happens.

If he can't make you come in such a short space of time, just whip out your vibrator, and hold it against your clitoris while he penetrates you – that should do the trick if nothing else does. And because orgasm is good for you – relaxing, gets all the blood galloping round your body and fills you with giggly well-being – you can return to work after your lunchtime liaison, entirely refreshed and happy. You don't get that from window-shopping.

noise

Long-term sex does partially rely on remembering to demonstrate that you still like each other. So even if you're coming violently on a regular basis, if you simply lie there while he goes through the familiar old routine and then emit a little whimper at the end of it, he may well start feeling

---

TIP

Make a rule that he can't initiate sex for two weeks – which puts just enough pressure on you to do it yourself. Men get sick of always being the ones to risk rejection – it hurts, baby – so it's lovely for him to feel that he is wanted after all. It doesn't take much – just once in a while, make the first move with a snog. Or given that most men like the direct approach, simply reach out and touch somebody by grabbing his penis under the bedclothes. Or on the bus, if you're feeling particularly frisky.

---

that he isn't quite the god of love you once thought he was. So, his performance will suffer accordingly, and he won't try as hard. So you'll be even less appreciative … and the same goes for him, too.

Yet it's so easy to raise your passion levels, and consequently his, without actually having an affair, or even pretending you're in a porn film. All you have to do is make more noise. Yes, it's a little embarrassing, it can't be denied. But come on, a few groans and gasps are all that's needed to make him feel like King Dong, and you – once you've got over feeling silly – will be much more in touch with what you're feeling, because you're reacting to every change of sensation, instead of just letting it happen.

He too should be vocal in his appreciation of whatever you're doing. Nobody wants a screamer – how many hotels have you stayed in, cursing the idiots in the next room who seem to think sex is supposed to be a five-cycle German opera? Nevertheless, totally silent sex is just unnerving – so moan and whimper all you like, and encourage him to do the same.

TIP

Men love to hear that you're appreciating their moves in bed – in fact, a survey found that 80% like noisy sex, and the other 20% probably live with their parents. If you lie there in deadly silence, he won't know whether you're loving every second or mentally doing the washing. So even if it doesn't come naturally, make a noise anyway – just begin with a little gasp or groan; you don't need to have hysterics to begin with. As you get used to expressing yourself, hysterics may come naturally, of course. If so, watch out for the neighbours. Thin walls are your worst enemy.

If both of you are comfortable with the idea of writing, then take turns to write an erotic story for each other to read. You can make it as pornographic or romantic as you like, depending on what style turns you on. The chances are yours will be all 'Desmond slipped the silken straps of Sophia's nightdress from her alabaster shoulders,' and his will say 'put it in me,' groaned Angel, 'I'm still wet from fucking Venusia all night, and now I want your hot tool'.

photo-me

Sound is one thing, accompanying visuals are quite another – and there are plenty of people who'd rather have their toenails removed with rusty pliers than commit their naked bodies to film. If you are one of them, don't agree to Polaroids or video, because you will automatically hate what you look like, and spend the rest of the evening/week/year arguing about why you should have plastic surgery immediately, which is not a basis for seductive conversation, really. Again, if you are someone who is fundamentally a worrier, you will be instantly convinced that once these Polaroids exist, your mother will stumble upon them, or that you'll die prematurely and they'll be auctioned amongst your personal effects, and all your friends and colleagues will come, weeping, to the auction, only to see 'Lot 224, Miscellaneous Photographs' flashed up on a giant projector screen. Or if you've got kids, that their innocence will be destroyed as they lisp, 'Mummy, why is daddy hurting you in the picture?' Or … anyway, you get the point. So only do this if you don't hate your body, are reasonably confident that you know a decent hiding place, and trust that your

---

TIP

Get yourself a Polaroid camera and have fun taking pictures of yourself in provocative poses – a picture of your breasts, or even bits,
can be enough to plummet him immediately into sexual mode –
well, with most men just walking down the street can do that, but
still. If you want to take a risk – and who doesn't, frankly? – then
tuck one into his jacket pocket for him to find while he's away from
you ... but perhaps you'd better leave a message telling him to do
that when he's alone. Unless you want all his colleagues getting a
good look at your Brazilian wax, that is.

---

partner won't dump you and post you on the internet (which is actually
the most realistic possibility).

If you are, however, you should definitely consider the Polaroid angle
on sex. Light yourself well (soft but direct, so you don't get weird shadows
that make you look like Ozzy Osbourne) and sit in the right position – sitting, your arms behind you so your breasts are thrust forward, stomach in,
shot three-quarters on, makes everyone look good, as does lying on your
side like the famous painting, *The Rokesby Venus*, because your waist automatically goes in and your legs are together, disguising less than perfect
thighs. If he wants to pose, be careful, as it's all too easy for men to look like
camp gay totty – try not to get him lying on his side looking smouldering,
it's a bit too 'Old Compton Street phone box' – but sitting up, playing with
his willy, is OK, or even standing up, but no hands on hips, alright, sailor?

The best way to feature both of you is to video yourselves – you
need to position a tripod at the end of the bed, focus the camera so the
whole bed is in shot, and then set it recording and make sure you stay

roughly within shot, as an entire tape of your joined calves and feet will not make riveting viewing, sexually speaking. You can get PC programmes that will let you edit the tape, if it's digital, and add music and even subtitles (well, you might want to pretend it's a French art-house movie – 'Veronique! It's my father, he has arrived prematurely from Paris!' 'Jean-Paul! I am also sleeping with your sister! Let's have a *pastis*,' et cetera). Alternatively, you may just want to watch the basic tape and enjoy actual porn starring your actual selves. It's a lot more exciting than actual porn starring large peroxide-haired Europeans, on the whole – but make sure you label the tape carefully – you really don't want to give your mates an extra special treat when they come round to watch *Gladiator*.

Spicing up your love life is well worth the effort – it may seem a little contrived or embarrassing at first, but if you persist, you'll forget that you were trying at all, because you'll be enjoying what you're doing so much. I'm convinced there'd be less affairs if there was more spicing up – it won't stop you fantasising about other people, admittedly, but it may well stop you doing anything about it.

5   sex toys

Some people believe that sex on its own should be enough, without the unnecessary addition of sex toys. All that vibrating, whizzing plastic in the bedroom? Not for the likes of us! Then they wonder why their sex lives are so dull and repetitive and why it takes them hours to come. The truth is, sex toys are a vitally useful tool in your armoury – not only do they provide you with an instant sex life should you happen to be single for a while, they also boost your sex life with a partner no end, as they can offer you the kind of thrills that normally you'd need a third person to administer – and your partner will almost certainly be grateful that you're getting your jollies from a bit of silicone, rather than his best mate.

Sex toys have come a long way from their rather shaky beginnings – whereas once they were sold as 'personal massagers' and required more technical know-how to wield than an AK47, you can now get pretty much any kind of sex toy that floats your personal boat, from revolving love-eggs to blow-up sheep. Though why a blow-up sheep would do so is something best kept to yourself, I suspect.

All the same, the old, miserable days of sneaking into filthy-looking 'Adults Only XXX' shops on dodgy streets, and plucking up the courage to ask for a vibrator that only came in one size and style – terrifying pink plastic – are long gone. Ann Summers led the way, but other entrepreneurs like the women-friendly sex shops Sh! In London and Gash in Sheffield, have made it infinitely easier for women to admit that sex toys are normal, fun, and not a badge of hideous shame. There are even upmarket sex

> **TIP**
>
> Vibrators are not just useful for genital stimulation – they're invaluable for locating your erogenous zones as well. Set it to 'low' and try it against your breasts, nipples, neck and inner thighs – in fact, try it anywhere that you suspect might be an erogenous zone and would like to check. It also works wonders for his balls. And don't ignore his nipples either – they still respond to vibration, as you will discover.

stores now – Coco de Mer and Myla, in London, cater for (doing-) It girls, who don't see anything extravagant about spending £700 on a crystal vibrator, or investing in a pretty *Toile de Jouy* nightdress which, on closer inspection, features beautifully designed cocks and vaginas. Sex toys have come out of the closet, and while they're still some way off being displayed on the coffee table (thankfully) they are more than acceptable purchases for the modern woman – and man. The only trouble is, there are so many types it'd be impossible to try them all. If you still can't face going into a shop and asking a real live assistant, even though they're seen it all before a hundred thousand times, you can order what you want over the Internet. It will arrive in plain packaging, and trust me, the postman will never know. Unless you decide to give him a private showing, that is.

sex toys for girls

Girls tend to do better when it comes to sex toys than men. That may be because sex toys for women are fun additions to a healthy sex life, or a handy way of having an orgasm when you're alone. For men, however, sex toys are often packaged as a weird substitute for a girlfriend – 'so real!',

'Wanda has an amazing 3-speed vagina,' and so on — which is just creepy in the extreme. If you;ve ever seen those odd-looking rubber fannies with horrible Sindy-doll hair coming out of plastic follicles, I'm sure you understand where I'm coming from. Still, they probably make a lot of men very happy, so best leave them to their world of fun with Inflatable Imogen, and concentrate on what sex toys can do for girls.

vibrators

There are thousands of different types of vibrator — but they all aim to do the same thing: to stimulate your clitoris and vagina, and smooth the path to orgasm. Some are so powerful they can make you come in seconds, others offer a more gentle journey, via a faint tingling sensation, which culminates in a few rhythmic contractions of the vagina, rather than the screaming, breathless helter-skelter that the really big hitters hope to give you. It's a nice idea to keep different types for different occasions, although as sex toys get more sophisticated, they offer different attachments and speeds in the same model. This is getting a little like selling motorbikes, and about as confusing, so let's get back to basics.

TIP

If he's using a vibrator on you — or you are, on his bum — it really helps to have some vocal guidance. Without any nerves, it's almost impossible for him to tell whether he's pushing too fast, or too hard — so if you can say 'that's perfect … bit further … stop there,' it will save him an awful lot of worry, trying to interpret whether your sharp intakes of breath meant 'oh, god, no!' or just 'oh yes! Yes!' And he should extend a similar courtesy to you, of course.

> **TIP**
>
> If vibrators are a whole new concept for you, start with a very little one – it doesn't need to be big and scary and phallic – you can get tiny lipstick-shaped ones that will cause no embarrassment whatsoever should they fall out of your bag. Unless someone wants to borrow your lovely shade of red, of course. But tiny ones are perfect for clitoral stimulation – there's no requirement to get a huge, veiny dildo that looks like the aftermath of King Dong's accident with a chainsaw. Start small – and if you like it, then hey, stay small.

Vibrators come either electricity-powered or battery-powered. If they require lots of whizzing, buzzing attachments, they may have a battery pack attached to them, or the battery might be one of the little disc-shaped integral ones. With cheaper models, the battery often fails to fit properly, which means you'll be seconds off the biggest orgasm of your life, when there's a little 'clunk' and you realise it's slipped sideways and the whole thing's just ground to a halt. The electric ones are safer – but you do need to plug them in, obviously, and on the down side, they really aren't terribly quiet.

Vibrators come in all manner of sizes – and shapes range from the discreet handbag-friendly mini-dildo kind to the enormous, throbbing, 14-inch sort that should probably only be used in the dressing rooms of heavy metal bands by trashed groupies. For everyone else, they're just too much to deal with. Certain men, particularly, get horribly insecure when confronted with giant vibrators, and begin to compare themselves most unfavourably with their plastic rivals. Reassure him all you like, but if you're unpacking Wayne the 12-inch Wonder-wand for the third time this week, he may have reason to be concerned. So don't start being unfaithful to him with your vibrator to the extent that you actually prefer it.

You can get vibrators that are disguised as anything but – from religious artefacts (one for all you lapsed Catholics out there) to giant corncobs to lipsticks. Most of them, however, do the same thing – which is to provide something to put inside your vagina that resembles a penis (lesbians often buy 'goddess' shaped vibrators to avoid this, but at the end of the day, they just resemble a penis with bad hair) and something to tickle your clitoris, which can be a separate attachment, or part of the wand itself, which you hold against yourself. Some prefer to run them up and down while they vibrate, others to hold them in the most sensitive place and wait for nirvana that way. Some even treat them like sports cars, flicking between speeds like Michael Schumacher flicks between gears.

Most vibrators are straight, but some are bendy, designed to reach the G-spot – and they probably do have a better chance of doing so than fingers. Natural Contours are a range which are shaped to fit your shape, and actually don't look like penises – they're curvy, come in different lengths, and nestle beautifully against your pubic mound.

The best-known vibrator is probably the Rabbit. It's G-spot friendly, with a rotating section full of little beads in the middle, and rabbit 'ears' to tickle your clitoris with. It's also a huge seller, having been featured on *Sex & The City* – and if it was good enough for Samantha …

love balls

Love balls are, in certain people's opinions – alright, that might just be mine – somewhat overrated. They are two little prickly spheres made of silicone, or the like, which are inserted into your vagina. Once there, they're supposed to roll about, stimulating as they go. But in truth, not only is it like trying to get a hedgehog's tampon up there, if you push them too far you can't feel a thing – as is the way with tampons – and if you don't, it feels like they're about to fall out. As, again, is the way with tampons. If you do manage to get them balanced somewhere acceptable, who knows, you might be beside yourself with excitement in no time – but I kind of doubt it.

butterfly

This is much more use – the Butterfly (though it goes under various other names) is a little vibrating disc which hooks over your hips like a pair of knickers. The idea then is, you put your knickers on over it to hold it in place against your clitoris, and off you go – orgasm as you go about your domestic duties, or attend high-level business meetings, or what-have-you. It's a very sexy idea, but in practice it could be a bit of a nightmare – you really don't need to be going all red and flushed as you enjoy Sunday dinner with your boyfriend's parents – unless his Dad's really that attractive, of course.

TIP

It is possible to buy sex toys such as the Butterfly with a remote-control attachment. So for a night out with a much more entertaining difference, stick the vibrating bit in your knickers, give him the controls, and off you go. Actually, the difference could be the screaming row you have when you hand him the controls and he turns the buzzer off just as you're about to come. That aside, as long as you know how to disguise the fact that you're turned on (and if you ever entertained boys at your parents' house, you probably do), go ahead – there's worse ways to liven up a Sunday night in the pub.

waterproof

Waterproof vibrators are ideal for the active woman caught in a rainstorm who fancies an orgasm to take her mind off the weather … or then again, they may simply be suitable for use in the bath and shower. This is a great idea, as for a lot of women the bathroom's the only place they're likely to get enough peace and quiet to masturbate – particularly if you live in a shared house, or have kids. You can purchase ones that are cunningly disguised to look like a sponge – put it between your legs in the bath or shower, and away you go; all the fun of an orgasm, none of the electrocution. In fact, do be careful – make sure it definitely is waterproof before you go ahead and jump in with it. What an embarrassing way to go, otherwise.

clit stimulators

The finger tickler is a thoroughly ingenious little device. It just looks like a baby splint – alright, it's not that sexy, but still … and it straps on to your finger – or his – which is then, of course, placed against the clitoris. So you get free access to your vagina, and lots of clitoral stimulation, without the unwieldy interference of a big dildo getting in the way.

TIP

It is possible to buy sex toys that exist mainly to encourage you to tighten your vaginal muscles. Obviously, should your partner buy you these, you must immediately stuff them up a different hole altogether, belonging to him. However, if it's your decision, then the tension required to hold them in place ensures that your PC muscles get a continual workout. Of course, there's always the worry that you'll forget and they'll drop out mid-tube train. Which would be bad.

> **TIP**
>
> For a vibrator on the cheap, you can't beat an electric toothbrush. Make sure no one's planning on using it to clean their teeth later, that's all. Aside from that, though, it works on exactly the same principle, and should deliver a similar thrill when it vibrates against your clitoris. If you like a little erotic abrasion, you can hold the bristles against yourself – but if, like most people, you think that sounds less fun than a bikini wax, just press the back of the head against your clitoris, an instruction that works well for oral sex, too.

dildos

And talking of dildos … they are just penis-shaped objects used in place of an actual penis. They're handy for anal penetration ('hello, vicar! So glad you could join us!') while he's inside you, or for using if his penis is having an off day, or he's just come three times and is exhausted. Some types are terrifying – dildos, not penises, though I do see what you mean – being enormous, 20-inch double-ended things. Now these are for double penetration and can suit both lesbians, and gay men, but if you fancy showing him exactly how anal penetration feels, they can be useful tools for the heterosexual couple too. Niiice!

condoms

Condoms are not, strictly speaking, a sex toy, admittedly. But they do come in all kinds of guises, which include French Ticklers. Possibly not a phrase used in the last 50 years, nevertheless, the condom with added bit – typically, a cockscomb, or a little bird, made of latex – are still available. The idea being that they reach the parts that penises cannot reach (that damned G-spot again) and stimulate it no end. This is based on the premise that he can actually roll on a condom that features a novelty penguin balancing on the tip, without collapsing in hysterics. A better bet, perhaps, are ribbed condoms, which actually are quite useful when it comes to creating friction – the basis of all sexual excitement. If you're very wet, his penis can go in so smoothly it's barely noticeable – but a ribbed condom slows the process down, and makes sure you feel him moving. Worth buying a pack, and much cheaper than plastic surgery.

diy

You can, of course, avoid purchasing any sex toys whatsoever and make do with whatever you have in your house. Clothes pegs for nipple clamps – plastic ones are less painful, be warned – or even paperclips, should you suddenly be overcome with an urge for a nipple-clamp whilst at the office.

For vibrators, the economy version is the electric toothbrush. Small, discreet and you can easily get it through customs without dying of embarrassment. You can even set your mobile phone to 'vibrate', and get all your friends to ring you up. But that is a bit of a stop-start option. Dildos are easier – there's always courgettes, bananas, aubergines (ow!), carrots, corn-on-the-cob … in fact, why are so many vegetables willy-shaped? There's a question.

Some women, I'm told, even use rounded-end deodorant bottles. But that's not terribly safe, being rather scratchy – and so embarrassing if it gets lodged up there.

sex toys for him

Sex toys for men are, as previously mentioned, not quite so varied and interesting as those aimed at women. Maybe that's because men are less likely to need help orgasming. Or maybe they just have less orifices to put things in. Well … they definitely do. Still, there are certain devices that can change a dull night into a fantastic one with the simple aid of a battery – or even just a bit of plastic.

cock rings

These are bendy little bits of plastic that fit round the base of his penis. The idea is that they retain his erection, and ensure that the maximum amount of blood fills it, keeping it hard and stiff. This increases the sensitivity for him, but is even better for you. Some cock rings even have attachments that rub your clitoris as he thrusts. In fact, this is just as much a sex toy for you as it is for him … still, who's complaining?

vibrators

Vibrators can do wonders for men, once they get over their occasional fears that using them is somehow girly. He should switch it to the strongest speed, and hold it against his penis – hey presto, instant erection – or put it on a lower setting and caress his balls with it. He can even push it into his anus, where it will do marvellous things, stimulating his prostate gland. The best kind of vibrator for a man is a fairly simply dildo-shaped or Natural Contours one, which you can trail over the tip of his penis, or hold alongside the shaft, splint-like, till he's all big and strong again. If you're feeling too lazy to give a hand job, it's a great way of turning him on, and you can use it while you give him a blow job, so long as you don't mind your mouth going all weird and tingly as a result. You can get cock rings that vibrate, but that may feel a little too much like being a food-processor for most men, and unless he has a deep urge to stick his penis into cake mix, it's perhaps best avoided.

anal beads

Rather like a rosary in appearance, anal beads do what they say on the tin – they're beads, and they go up his arse. The idea is that you push them up there, leave a little thread hanging out, and just as he's about to orgasm, you pull them out with a theatrical flourish, and give him a titanic orgasm of epic proportions, due to the sudden effect of the rushing movement on his prostate. You will, of course, be using lubrication, should you attempt this – and you will not shout 'oh my god, I just thought, they might have pooh on!' at the crucial moment. Not unless you want to give him sexual hang-ups for the rest of his life you won't, at any rate. You can even get Anal Sticks, which do much the same thing – and if you're of a craft-making disposition, you can even make your own! But make sure they're tightly tied on, you really don't want to be explaining to the nurse why he's got half a Guatemalan bracelet up his arse.

blow up!

Let's just clarify now, we're only including blow-up dolls for the sake of thoroughness … it's extremely unlikely that he'll be attempting to introduce one into your love-making sessions. We hope. However realistic – and these days, the expensive ones are scarily like having sex with a Californian starlet, even down to the plastic content and conversational ability – they are basically the Choice of The Odd Loner, so if he does suggest that Silicone Suzy joins you in the boudoir, you're fully at liberty to stick a pin in her thigh and watch her crumple.

sex gloves

These are simply gloves with different textures on the fingers – and again, if you were feeling of a craft-fair bent, you could make your own, though they may be hard to sell at the local WI jamboree. They may have one finger fur, one leather, one lace, one rubber … you get the idea. So you just try out each one on his skin, and see which produces the best effect. Hopefully not fur, or you'll be out trapping bears to turn him on before you know it. Leather's always a good bet – so maybe Dad's driving gloves could be put to a whole new purpose…

mints

Sex shops sell all kinds of liquids that you're supposed to paste on and lick off – 'willy growing lotion,' 'booby drops,' you know the kind of thing. And they're weirdly flavoured, in that whatever flavour they claim to be they all taste like gone-off wine gums. However, you can enjoy a much more pro-found effect simply with an extra-strong mint. Just suck one for a while, and then lick and suck his penis. The effect will be instant – not quite pain, but enough stimulation to make all his nerve endings start firing like the charge of the light brigade. If it hurts, alternate with mouthfuls of water. Don't get carried away and rub the mint directly onto his skin – unless you really, really hate him, of course.

diy

There are, once again, a variety of household objects that lend themselves to pleasing his penis no end. Fruit and vegetables aren't quite so perfect as they are for you, of course, because not many are vagina-shaped – though he could have a go with a fig, there is something vaguely distasteful about the whole idea of it. So your best bet is to eat fruit off his penis (see

Chapter 4 for details) and save the vegetables for anal penetration – 'more stew, Mum?' – if that's what he fancies. Small vegetables, mind, there's no point in being needlessly cruel.

You can also use items that give him new sensations – feathers trailed along his penis and used to tickle his balls will provide a fantastic thrill for him, and he can always return the favour on your inner thighs. You can use a feather duster if you wish, but it's a little bit Ken Dodd for some tastes. A simple ostrich feather (what do you mean you don't have any lying around?) should suffice.

There are certain things you can wrap round his penis when you're giving him a hand job that will ensure spectacular orgasm – chief of these is a pearl necklace. As well as being slang for him coming all over your breasts, the real thing can produce sensations that your hand just isn't capable of giving him.

You just wrap your string of pearls – and of course fake ones are just as good – round his penis as many times as they'll go, then put your hand over them and proceed with the normal style of hand job. The feeling of the little bumps rubbing all over his penis is highly erotic – but if you don't want him to ejaculate all over Granny's pearls, make sure you whip them away in plenty of time.

You can try the same effect with silk scarves, wooden beads, pieces of fun fur, crisp packets … actually, maybe not crisp packets. But anything else painless and sexy to the touch is worth a try.

sex toys during sex

So far, the whole idea has revolved around taking turns: you do something, then he does something to you. But some sex toys come into their own during sex itself, and you can both share them. The best way is to hold a vibrator in between you during sex, so it's pressing on your clitoris and his balls at the same time. Alternatively, you can hold it against his balls and anus while he thrusts into you, or lie so it's angled at your own anus – or inside it – while he's inside your vagina. Vibrators can also be rubbed across your breasts, or his nipples – in fact, the only thing it's really not worth doing with one is attempting to snog it.

games & props

Playing sexual games is a great way to introduce a little more fun into your sex life without joining a swingers' society. They are particularly good for slightly inhibited people, as the games' rules dictate what you have to do – effectively, as long as you go along with the rules, you have no say in the matter, which frees you up nicely to be as outrageous as you want.

strip poker ... and the rest

Strip-games are the perfect way to begin a sex session. Especially with someone you'd like to have sex with but are too shy to actually make a move on. Strip poker is only one version – and if you're not sure of the rules, the beauty of this game is that the strip part can be adapted to almost any other competitive game. Strip Monopoly might take a really long time, though. What you want, ideally, is a game that will result in great, sweeping reversals of fortune, allowing forfeits and tension to come into it as well. Something like 21, or Blackjack, are good card games to try – that way it's all in the hands of fate, rather than reliant on your own skill.

If you find the clothes are coming off too fast, and you want to prolong the simmering sexual tension, then simply add forfeits to the mix –

sexual ones, of course. He might have to lick your nipples for one minute, or you might have to masturbate in front of him – anything to crank up the desire between you, without actually fulfilling it. And the game lasts as long as you can bear it to.

blindman's buff

You take turns to be blindfolded. Whoever can see conceals a small item somewhere about their naked person, and the blindfoldee has to locate it. The amusing twist on this one is, that he or she can only search with their mouth, so kissing, licking and nibbling are all allowed; touching is not. It goes without saying that the hider will become increasingly sophisticated when it comes to where the item is hidden – although it does count as cheating to keep moving it. Suggested items are a chocolate button, or a raspberry – nothing that can be choked on, at any rate. And when it's found, you swap roles. Or rip off the blindfold and make mad, passionate love – whichever comes first.

porn charades

This is extremely simple, yet strangely effective. All you have to do is act out whatever you'd like to have done to you, without actually speaking. So if you want to be taken from behind, you simply adopt the doggy position, and thrust your bum in the air. But it's more complicated if you also want him to caress your clitoris at the same time, with a vibrator. And if he wants to stand in front of a mirror, watching you masturbate, how's he going to get that across without props … Play it naked, and when anyone guesses correctly, they get to do it for real. If they don't it's the other player's go. A word of warning though – it's not one for family gatherings.

porn snap

Again, simple – you simply hire a porn video, and every time the actors do something, you do it too. It helps not to rent one about a gang bang though, unless you have a really strong relationship. Ideal are ones featuring hilariously unattractive models, so neither of you gets jealous. You just keep an eye on what's happening, and follow the leaders on screen. It should give you an entertaining sexual work-out, at the very least. And if you see her deep-throating him and wonder what her secret is? Don't worry, it's just camera trickery. It doesn't really happen unless you're a sword-swallower, and that is not a game I'd recommend.

fantasy and role play

Fantasy deserves a whole book to itself – as Nancy Friday proved with her series featuring women's and men's deepest erotic thoughts. Your fantasies are your business, and there's no law that says you have to share them with your partner – besides, he may not want to know your most private thoughts about zoo-keepers and the like. And you may not really wish to delve too thoroughly into his issues with his ex-girlfriend and a jar of marmite. However, shared fantasies are an entirely different kettle of fish (though if he's fantasising about one, stop right there, nobody wants to know).

If you have the courage to tell each other what turns you on, you're opening up a whole new chapter of your shared sexuality, which can unleash feelings you never knew you had, and clear the way for some fantastic experiences. Because once you've opened up, and made sure he isn't reeling in horror, you can then enact your fantasies in real life. That's 'enact,' notice, not 'live out' – which is an entirely different thing. Pretending to be a hooker is a long way from standing on the ring-road with no knickers on, eyeing up lorry drivers.

And pretending he's a wicked headmaster and you're a naughty schoolgirl is a very long way indeed from the dreadful court case that would ensue should he try it for real.

When it comes to discussing your fantasies, particularly those you'd like to act out, it pays to go easy at first – there's nothing worse than one's partner breathing 'you what?' in disgust and horror, before flinging back the duvet and going to cry in the bathroom. So leave out all references to any of his friends or family members you've always fancied, never mention exes, and go easy on the whole Brad Pitt thing, specially if he looks nothing like him whatsoever.

Suitable fantasies for sharing will generally include a role for each other – so if you'd like to be a lap dancer, let him be the paying punter, or if you fancy being a saucy businesswoman, allow him to be the nervous interviewee for the post of your assistant. The same goes for him – if he'd like to be the Lord of the Manor, you can be the housemaid, or the PVC-clad dominatrix to his trembling love-slave. It's vital that you're both happy with the roles you're assigned, and you aren't both striving for power at the expense of the game – 'No! I'm the Roman Emperor! You're just a slave!' 'Piss off! I thought of it in the first place!' doesn't make for great sex.

Once you've decided on your scenario, however, you'll need to get some props together to help you make the scene vaguely convincing. Look, it doesn't need to be all that convincing, you just have to make it faintly believable for the duration of foreplay and sex – no one's going to be asking the director about their motivation or anything, calm down.

Useful props to have are: a cape (works for evil headmasters, super-heroes, vampires, Florence Nightingale – alright, I know, some people are just a bit unusual in their tastes) and dominatrixes, very tarty high heels (works for everything, but particularly hookers and lap dancers), glasses (works for the business interview because you can remove them from each other at the crucial moment), suits (good for business, again – also, in his case, a high-class escort's customer), pearls (see above, also ideal for Lady Chatterley types), an apron and white hat (good for nurses and maids), and a peaked cap (chauffeurs, policemen, er, traffic wardens … well, maybe if you're into S&M and like to administer punishment, it could work).

Of course you can supplement your dressing-up box with whatever else you want: Bruce Willis-style white vests, firemen's helmets, lady-in-distress nighties … whatever suits your particular fantasies – even if that's a rubber gimp mask and a pair of marabou-trimmed slippers. Hey, listen, if it works for you …

erotica

Sex toys, games and props can all be helped along by a little sprinkle of one final thing – no, not drugs, you at the back – erotica, which includes books, films and magazines. Indeed, you may call it porn if you wish, but we're not necessarily talking about hardcore action. Books such as the *Black Lace* series, aimed at women – but almost certainly read by men – are perfect erotica, in that they contain a storyline, and characters who aren't simply vessels for sperm – but at the same time they do spend most of their lives shagging in a variety of interesting and challenging new ways. The books are perfect for you to read before he arrives in bed – thus bringing you to the level of sexual arousal that men tend to simmer at most of the time – or for you to read to each other.

Magazines, too, have their place – in your house that might be 'on a bonfire,' but bear with me. The market has expanded, in a bid to fight the encroaching porn-provision of the Internet, and the newer magazines are aiming themselves at couples, with literate writing, and photo shoots of gorgeous people in interesting positions, rather than the usual dimwit teen in a split beaver pose, which may not, understandably, appeal. Erotica allows you to explore the sides of your sexuality you've kept under wraps – your secret fantasies about women, say, or his occasional thoughts about group sex – and brings it into the open in a non-threatening way.

Porn films too are worth considering as an erotic tool – it is possible to buy the kind that are made with women in mind nowadays, which may actually feature some kind of plot, and a heroine who sometimes has fully-formed thoughts before she opens her legs. If all that sounds way too scary and hardcore, consider erotic books – Anais Nin, Erica Jong, even D.H. Lawrence have all written literature that has been, in its day, considered obscene. Now, however, it's considered classic, and you could happily read it on the tube. Or, better still, in bed.

6 adventurous sex

Adventurous sex suggests you're doing it on some mosquito-infested bank somewhere in Borneo, or up K2 with only a sleeping bag between you and certain death. However, you can have wildly adventurous sex without going further than the bedroom – and besides, sex on K2 is frightfully dull. I know, I've tried it. (Obviously, this is a lie.)

Adventurous sex is all about pushing the boundaries, trying things you've never done before – and possibly, things you wouldn't tell your friends, should they ask. Well, you've got to have some secrets, haven't you? We're not talking about dodgy, risky, picking up strangers sex – you go right ahead if you like that, but I refuse to take the blame when it turns out he was an escaped convict/

TIP

Magazines always bang on about the hot/cold blow job, which is, ultimately, just slightly painful and not that much fun, given that most versions seem to involve you taking alternate sucks of ice and chilli. But if you simply sip on a chilled glass of white wine, and then nibble a bit of ginger, it'll be far less unpleasant – for both of you. And he'll still get the remarkable sensations of heat and cold on his willy. He can return the favour, but not quite as hot and not quite as cold – you're more sensitive, see?

mad/emotionally stunted. We are, however, talking about dodgy, risqué, picking up your partner and whirling him over your head sex.

Anything you can think of that two (or more) people can do sexually without getting arrested, indeed, counts as adventurous sex. At the very least, it probably involves leaving the lights on.

anal sex

And we're straight in at the deep end with every man's fantasy. Well, not strictly every man – probably just 99.9% and the .1% are scared it'll make them gay. They'd like to if they weren't so uptight … Men love it, you see, because not only is it forbidden, and therefore thoroughly dirty – in the best sense of the word – it's also a fantastically tight fit, because the anus is not meant to accommodate a baby, it's only meant to accommodate … well, yes, anyway. So it's a lot smaller, has no natural lubrication, and basically offers the most fantastic, friction-packed experience on a man's penis

---

TIP

If you're going to have anal sex, bear in mind that while it's not dangerous, it isn't specifically what the anus is designed for, shall we say … So if you make a habit of it, you are putting yourself in some danger of stretching and pain, and well, you'd have to have a lot of anal sex with giant marrows, but ultimately, you may end up with anal muscles that work slightly less effectively, which equals incontinence. Argh! So to avoid all that, the best advice is to limit it to once every few weeks – and if you can't sit down the next day, that's probably more than enough.

> **TIP**
>
> When you're already stimulated, you're more relaxed, so it's easier for him to slide a finger into your anus. It still helps to use lubrication, though, and go slowly. If he pushes a finger in while he's got another in your vagina, the combined pressure can be much more stimulating than just anal penetration by itself. Moving his fingers with a slow in-and-out rhythm should provide an exciting sensation around your G-spot, too.

that he could wish for without forking out for a team of highly-trained rent boys with the internal muscle control of cocaine traffickers. So no wonder he likes it. For girls, however, the experience may not provide quite such a winning scenario. Whilst some absolutely love it, because of its naughty nature, and the knock-on stimulating effect on their vaginas, a lot of girls think of anal sex as slightly less fun than pooing a giant carrot would be. And the initial sensation is not that dissimilar, it has to be said. So if you are going to give him the chance to fulfil this particular lifetime ambition, there's a few things you should know first. Most importantly, whatever you believe about your bowels prolapsing, it's not true. You'd have to be having a hell of a lot of anal sex, with a hell of a lot of big dicks, for that to even be an option. And assuming you're not, have no fear, your anus will spring back into its normal tiny shape soon afterwards. So if that's the kind of thing you spend a lot of time worrying about, be reassured.

Secondly, if you are going to do it, you need to be very well lubricated around there. It will bloody hurt if you try it from a standing start, believe me. A generous helping of KY should do, unless you're so wildly aroused you can generate enough yourself to do the job – but even so, on this occasion, the wetter the better, to be brutally frank. Beforehand, he should have made sure to spend enough time on foreplay to relax you entirely – it's no good assuming the position and hissing 'go on then, get it over with' through gritted teeth. Well, you can, but that may kill the atmosphere to be honest.

He should also make sure to use a condom – the skin of the anus is not made for friction, and tears very easily, so any diseases can gallop right into your bloodstream and make hay. It's also not the most sterile environ-ment for him to be sticking his penis in either – so you may as well err on the side of caution with this one. The best position for anal sex – and I'm sure your Mother will already have told you this – is doggy style. But don't thrust your bum as high as you would with ordinary doggy – you really don't want penetration that deep, because until you're used to it, it will be a squeeze at best and agonising at worst. He must push very gently – regardless of how excited he is – until the tip has penetrated your anus. If you find you've clenched up with nerves, don't panic, just allow him to use his fingers to very gently massage and stretch the hole slightly. He can insert

---

TIP

If you feel compelled to rim – remember that thing where you lick each others' bottoms, like little doggies – the only thing that's really important is to be clean, because the bot is a breeding ground for odd bacteria, which is fine when bottom-bound but not so good in your mouth. It's a good idea to keep a pack of wet wipes by the bed, so you can just whisk it over your bits, should the urge to lick where the sun don't shine overtake you. And if you can overcome your natural inhibitions, it can feel fantastic, so it's definitely worth the price of a wipe.

TIP

Reassuringly, anal sex toys all have a little flange, which stops them disappearing up inside, and prevents accident and emergency staff being harassed nightly by herds of humiliated men, all with plastic dildos wedged up their bums. So if you want specific toys for anal penetration, make sure you get the ones that state what they're for and have taken this into account in their design. It's a lot easier for stuff to disappear up arses than up vaginas – hence the number of hilarious nurses' tales, about light bulbs, cucumbers, hoovers … and as far as I know, hoovers don't come with a flange.

one finger first, followed by two – if he gets carried away and keeps going until he's inserting whole marrows, though, that's the time to ask questions.

Once he's able to get it in – and if he is the proud owner of a really, really big penis, he may have to accept that he never will, as this is the one time having a small one is a positive advantage – he should go slooooowly. Just push it a couple of inches in, and almost come out again. If at this point, you are shouting 'ooow!' then perhaps it's not going to happen tonight. If you're merely thinking 'hmm, what a bizarre and strangely exciting feeling,' then you may go right ahead. If you can take it, he can thrust gently in as far as feels comfortable – not for him, he's having a whale of a time – for you. The problem will come when he's well on the way to orgasm, and is tempted suddenly to speed up dramatically, and thrust in a downright reckless fashion, which may well translate into downright painful. So he must be constantly vigilant that he isn't getting carried away and hurting you. Of course, there's a chance that you too may be getting carried away and shouting 'go, go, go!' in which case go ahead. But don't blame me when you can't sit down tomorrow.

You can have anal sex in any position – but the other one that works well is you bending over the table, as it provides easy access to the correct hole for him, and gives you something to brace yourself against. Missionary position is rubbish for anal sex, don't even attempt it. But if you do the table thing, don't tell the relatives what you were doing on it last night when they arrive for Sunday lunch. And you can go on top – but it's hard to get it in from that angle, so don't be surprised if it all ends in collapse.

Just to be sensible for a moment, he mustn't penetrate your vagina after he's been in your anus, as that's a very handy way to transfer tons of bacteria over that you really don't want in there. Other than that, go ahead. He can penetrate you with a dildo while you have anal sex if that appeals, or you can penetrate him with said dildo, he can have his fingers inside you at the same time as he's penetrating your anus ... oh, my dears, the possibilities are endless. Ish.

Of course, the irony is, his anus features a prostate gland, which makes anal penetration an absolute party in the park for him. You, however, have no prostate. Still, life's a funny thing, eh?

TIP

Men have more testosterone, which thickens their skin – and because women have less and therefore thinner skin, generally, women can take less pain. This is worth remembering whatever you're doing, but particularly relevant when it comes to S&M. What feels like a stimulating slap to him can be an agonising blow to her – so if he is wielding the cane, he needs to make sure he's being careful, and letting you set the pace.

> **TIP**
>
> If you're going to spank each other with a cane, choose it with care – the last thing you want is great red weals all over your arse. Half the eroticism, too, is in the swishing motion – hearing it whisk through the air builds the excitement before it strikes, and a great big wooden stick won't do that – but a small, bendy one will. Have a practice first with a garden cane, and based on how much pain you find a turn-on – if any – buy a cane that's thicker or thinner, accordingly.

sado masochism

Sadism is named after the Marquis de Sade, who enjoyed inflicting pain. And Masochism is named after Baron Sacher-Masoch, who enjoyed receiving it. Obviously, the two would have been a perfect pairing, but sadly they never met. Most couples, however, who favour a little SM activity tend to take the opposing roles – it's rare to find serious S&M-ers who take it in turns because when giving or receiving pain or control forms a large part of somebody's sexuality, it tends to err in a certain direction. For those who are merely playing, though, it's entirely possible to swap roles around, and try personas on for size.

One of you is dominant, one submissive. It isn't necessarily about inflicting actual pain on your partner – S&M can be as mild as being blindfolded and doing his or her bidding. But it can be as strong as being whipped, hung from a harness, or strapped and handcuffed, being beaten with a cat o' nine tails. Exploring deeply into the world of S&M requires a great deal of trust in each other, and total understanding of what is and isn't too dangerous to experiment with. And as this is not the S&M hand-

> **TIP**
>
> If dressing up in tight rubber appeals, it pays to know that getting into it is like struggling into a full-body condom. That is, difficult, painful, and not remotely erotic. But a way of making it easier to slide on without catching yourself painfully is with liberal applications of talc, which smoothes over all your lumps and bumps beautifully. Getting out of it, however is a different matter – and unless you want to crush his 'mystery woman' fantasy totally, you might want to do this in private.

book, for our purposes we'll assume you don't have a huge fetish, and that you simply fancy a bit of leather-based love-life-spicing.

dressing the part

The easiest way to start your journey into the world of pain and pleasure (or at least, fluffy handcuffs) is with the dress code. S&M-ers like leather, rubber, and PVC, all fabrics that mould to the body, feel like skin, only with a harder edge, and carry a suggestion of restraint – most garments either expose a lot of flesh, or are extremely tight and figure-revealing, with bondage straps, studs and shiny bits. The look is, of course, highly sexy on women – most men take one look and think 'Michelle Pfeiffer. Catwoman. Yesss!' even if you look more like Tina Turner in *Mad Max*. On men, however, it's slightly less than hot, unless he gets it absolutely right – and studded PVC posing pouches don't work for many men, it has to be said. Wait, make that 'any'. He might just about get away with leather trousers and motorbike boots – though he may only attain 'hairdresser out clubbing' – and a studded belt, a dog collar and leather gloves might be acceptable too. The full rubber gimp-mask look, however, is best saved for the hardcore fan. A long, black leather coat makes any man look like Steve McQueen, and a few chains – particularly through his nipples – should complete the 'S&M Lite' look.

For you, high heels are essential – ideally, shiny thigh-high boots covered in buckles. Sex shops sell vast ranges of leather, metal and stud-encrusted clothing, most of which has special holes for breasts and willies. So don't be shy.

s&m accessories

If you're committed to the S&M thing, you'll need a few props – chief of which is handcuffs. Handcuffs are ideal for pinning you down so you can't wriggle away (as countless policemen have discovered over the years.) They are, though, easy to use wrongly – and pulling your hands behind your back and cuffing them there is painful after only a couple of minutes, not to mention stupidly uncomfortable. You should have your wrists handcuffed to the headboard of the bed – or the nearest piece of heavy furniture. Your arms should be above your head, but not stretched so hard you're popping your shoulder joints out of place with every movement –

TIP

When you're tying each other up, it's useful to use restraints you can actually undo afterwards. Which is why anything with nylon in it is a really bad idea, and silk or cotton is fine. Using discarded stockings, then, while a dirtily attractive notion, is a disaster in reality, because the lycra tightens to a flesh-choking grip, and the knots are impossible to unpick. The best bet is silk scarves.

---

make sure there's some bend in your elbows. You can get ankle cuffs too, to pin each leg to the end of the bed – all of which relies on you having some kind of old Victorian brass bed – so if you haven't, you'd better sell yours and buy one, hadn't you?

There are even special sheets you can purchase with integral foot and wrist straps, but in all honesty they do make you look like something out of *One Flew Over The Cuckoo's Nest*, so don't invest in one unless you have some Jack Nicholson/Nurse Ratched fantasy thing going on, OK?

You may also like to purchase a little whip, or a cat o' nine tails – which is a little whip with tiny leather strands coming out of it, which gives a softer swish to the buttocks. You don't have to whack the living crap out of your partner with it, just give them a tingly little slap on the bum. And a back-hand stroke gives you a better angle for a smooth whip than a forward stroke, though you can alternate the two, back and forth, like an angry ping-pong player. There's a little whisk-y one you can buy, called The Flogger – it gives a sharp sensation without actually causing untold damage – so that's the kind of thing you should be investigating if you're really serious.

You can buy custom-made blindfolds, all lovely and leather – or you

---

TIP

If you want to try bondage but handcuffs seem a bit hardcore, you can buy bondage tape from sex shops – like gaffer tape, but not nearly as hard to unpeel, it simply wraps round your ankles or wrists without causing pain, and can be pulled off or snipped off when you've finished. You can use it as a gag, theoretically – but gagging can be a dangerous move, so go easy and don't wrap it round each other's heads six times or anything.

> **TIP**
>
> You can get leather dog-collars and leads to drag your sex-slave around behind you – and wear them to a private club (no, not the local Conservative Association, you fool) or simply play Master and Servant at home. If you do, though, be extra-vigilant about how much force you're using – power-games can tap into all sorts of buried emotions, and you don't want to be getting off on the fantasy, only to turn round and find he's sobbing because of his unresolved issues. So go easy.

can just make do with his woolly arsenal scarf if that seems a bit of a wild extravagance. Or compromise with a silk one.

Of course for the serious S&M-er, there's a vast range of equipment, from rubber coffins to tapes of white noise intended to disorient masochist love-slaves. But hopefully, that end of the market will not be troubling you.

what to do

The association of pain with pleasure is a complex one, and while some find any kind of stimulation arousing, others may hate the sensation of experiencing pain during sex. The theory is that when you're aroused, you're filled with endorphins, which enable you to undergo stronger sensations than you'd normally withstand – but that doesn't mean you have to like having your bum spanked. And just in case you don't, but your partner's lost in a world of flaring nostrils and cracking whips, those clever S&M people have come up with a code that means 'stop.'

In S&M games, 'No' can mean all kinds of things. It can mean 'Oh my god! Yes! Yes! no! I'm so excited!' Or it can mean 'No! I'm pretending to be a virgin you're deflowering! Don't stop!' Or ... well, it can mean all sorts of other things if you're role-playing. So to make sure that if your handcuffs are starting to chafe painfully, or your whipping isn't going according to plan, you use the traffic-light code instead. If you want to stop, you say 'Red!' – there's no other context you could use this word in, so he – or you – will immediately know what you mean. And if you're worried he might stop, you simply shout 'green!' for 'go ahead with what you're doing'. Presumably, if you quite like it but you don't want him to get completely carried away, you say 'amber.' Now there's passionate!

blindfolding

When you're blindfolded, you are basically in the submissive role. You have no control over what's going on – and if you're tied up as well, you're about as powerful as a day-old kitten. So unless you're very experienced at this game, don't use gags, because it's extremely tempting to have a major-league panic once you realise you can't speak or see. A kidnapping scenario might sound like good, dangerous fun before you start, but games of con-

---

TIP

DIY S&M is a whole lot easier to sort out than the kind where you have to explain to a spotty teenage assistant exactly what you want to do with that rubber diving suit. And S&M props can be found around the house ... try tight rubber washing-up gloves for a different hand-job sensation, plastic pegs for nipple clamps (yes, you may look daft, but think of the money you're saving), and a soft hair-brush for a little light spanking.

> **TIP**
>
> If you have a fantasy that you want to confess to your partner, but you don't know how he'll react, find an erotic story that deals with the theme (and if you can't find one, OK, maybe you're a little unusual …) and leave it lying around in the loo. Then later ask if he happened to see it, and what he thought of it. If he says 'oh my god, that's so perverted! Some people beggar belief,' then perhaps it's best left a private fantasy. But if he says 'fwooar, that's a bit horny,' then you might just be in.

trol can have quite deep emotional effects, and bring out all kinds of buried fears you never knew you had. You should tread carefully with it, and don't ever do anything you're not convinced is a great idea. So leave the gags to the professionals (Bernard Manning, Bob Monkhouse … no, not that sort of gag, they're too dangerous and horrible to even contemplate) and make sure you're able to speak.

harness

You can buy devices that give you the full dungeon effect in your own home, without actually needing to kit out the cellar like a *News of the World* exposé. Harnesses that fit over doors, for instance, which work like handcuffs but mean that you're hanging slightly off the floor – like a 17th-century prisoner – lend themselves to whipping and spanking games. I can't say it works for me, but hey, if you like the idea of being suspended by your wrists while your partner flogs you, go ahead, make your day. There are also harnesses which hold you in a position for easy access – your legs are parted and your arms are pinned down by the ankle and

TIP

You may be of the belief that you'll look like a common hooker in a peephole bra and crotchless panties, but the only possible response to this is 'so?'. You will look unbelievably hot, and by presenting what you're offering in such an appealing and upfront fashion, you are basically telling him that you find him so attractive you want to show yourself off to the best advantage. It's much naughtier than straight nudity, and once in a while it doesn't hurt to get a little dirty – plus it means that if you're a bit lazy, you get to have sex without getting undressed.

wrists straps that they feature – and submission is definitely the name of the game in one of these.

handing over control

You may find, if you take turns being dominant and submissive, that you both fall naturally into certain roles – which are often the opposite of your normal roles in the relationship. Powerful men, for instance, often like to be controlled sexually because it means they can hand over responsibility – and the same goes for women who wield power in normal life. Which makes you wonder what Mrs Thatcher and Denis used to get up to ... but let's not go there, eh? It helps to decide on your scenario in advance – you don't have to go as far as writing a script, but having a vague idea of whether you're being Sub or Dom, and what the idea behind the scene is, makes it more convincing and enjoyable. Partly because it seems a bit silly to finish your tea, watch *EastEnders*, and then say, 'right, shall we go upstairs and whip each other senseless now?' Having a plot – however shaky and ill-thought-out – gives you more reason to be doing it, and helps you to shed your inhibitions more effectively. Even if it gets no further than 'you've been a very naughty boy, now bend over.' Useful scenarios include dungeon master/mistress and prisoner, virgin and evil tyrant, lord of darkness and slave ... come on, it's not that difficult, is it?

If actual whipping seems a little harsh, there's no reason why you shouldn't give spanking a try. It's easier to control pain levels that way, as he – or you – can feel exactly how hard a hand is slapping bare arse, whereas with a cat o' nine tails you're not going to feel a thing except crazed with power. If it does get a little too painful, it's worth keeping some body lotion in the fridge, and rubbing it on the red bits for a tingly sensation of relief, and, could it be ... ah, yes! Must be arousal ...

After a certain period of time – could be ten minutes, could be hours – the game will almost always result in sex. But S&M-ers like to tease their partner to the point of orgasm, and then back away without letting them come – which is another form of mild torture. Eventually you'll be allowed your reward, but deferring the pleasure makes it even more enjoyable when it finally happens.

TIP

Don't be shy about trimming your pubic hair – there's nothing wrong with it the way it is, but it's pleasant to have a neat little triangle. And why stop there ... you can trim it into a heart or a tiny Brazilian-waxed strip, which appeals to men reared on porn. Hell, snip it into a parallelogram for fun if you want to – but don't ignore the whole area till Sleeping Beauty's forest is travelling down your thighs; it's sexier to keep it outside of the thigh area ...

TIP

When you're dressing up, the idea is to keep at least some of your clothes on during sex – and as you will almost certainly be wearing stockings and suspenders, the vital thing to know is that you always put knickers on over suspenders. I can't tell you the amount of trouble caused by couples wrestling with resistant elastic in a bid to expose enough flesh to actually have sex with each other – all because she put her knickers on first. Discard the rest of the cheeky nurses' uniform if you must (must you?), but please, it's vital that you keep on your shoes and stockings … at least for a while.

---

clubs

For the committed S&M-er, there's a whole social scene out there – and hey, who'd want to miss out on that? There are specialist shops devoted to the pastime, selling all kinds of accoutrements, whips, chains, and leather and rubber goods. And even more excitingly, there are social clubs devoted to aficionados of pain and pleasure.

But if you attend these members-only extravaganzas, you have to be prepared to see stuff that's hard to forget – couples whipping each other, naked and in public, group sex in giant spiders' webs, people hanging from manacles wearing rubber hoods … just like Sunday lunch at mum's, really. If you want to watch without joining in, it may be OK for a while – but unless your club welcomes voyeurs, you may be expected to get down and dirty yourselves. So be prepared.

watersports

Watersports are adventurous sex and then some. Well, some might say adventurous, others might just recoil in horror murmuring, 'how could you?' Most of us, we can admit, are probably of Group Two – because being peed on just doesn't do it for us. However, who are we to judge? And if you like the idea of being weed on, or weeing on someone else, you have every right to give it a whirl. The main attractions to devotees are the total lack of inhibition, the naughtiness of doing something forbidden, and the sensation of warmth and wetness it entails. Also, the urethra can become aroused if stimulated, so if he's playing with the hole, the urge to actually wee could be overwhelming, so it's reassuring to know he won't run for the hills, should you let it happen.

If you do, make sure you're doing it on a large plastic sheet. The lounge carpet will never recover otherwise. Have a mop and bucket to hand, so the smell isn't an issue (unless that turns you on … oh dear) and drink plenty of water beforehand so your wee is a healthy straw colour

TIP

Coming in your face is seen by some women as degrading – but if you're going to sit on his, it seems only fair. They love it because accepting his semen all over you is tantamount to saying 'I want the very essence of your manhood' (or as he might put it, 'yes! I want your hot come all over me, big boy!'. Either way, it's a sexy thing to do because it implies total acceptance. Kind of like if he let you talk about shoes for a full hour when a match report's on the radio. And it's only sperm – you can always wash it off.

and relatively clean. Drinking wee is a really bad idea, whatever a bunch of alternative old hippies may think – so try to avoid that if possible. Apart from that, do whatever comes naturally, which tends to be one lying down and one standing up – or crouching – and doing the weeing. And hey, you kids enjoy yourselves, y'all hear?

threesomes & group sex

Here we come to the really risky bit of adventurous sex. It's all very well having fantasies about sleeping with another woman, or with two men – but if you decide to put it into practice, a warning siren should go off, and people in white protection suits should commence running up and down, spraying giant extinguishers and shouting, 'Clear the building! Clear the building!' That's how dangerous it is. I'm not talking about nasty diseases – though that can be a worry. I'm talking about emotional nuclear meltdown. Jealousy is a powerful and vengeful god, and if you give it half a chance it can ruin your relationship – you know, the one you thought was totally secure? That one.

TIP

Mutual masturbation – which in this case means masturbating in front of each other – can be a big turn-on for both of you, as well as highly educational, because it shows you exactly what each other likes. It takes a little courage to get going, but once you do, holding each other's gaze can be one of the sexiest things you'll ever do. If that feels too intimate, video each other masturbating alone, and watch the tapes together – believe me, no one will be embarrassed.

> **TIP**
>
> Watching other people have sex can be a real turn-on, but obviously, not that many people are up for it. You can, however, buy videos featuring actual, real people banging away at each other – renowned director Ben Dover also favours the unsophisticated porn technique, and makes films of ordinary-looking folk having a bunk-up in lighting that wouldn't disgrace the average butcher's shop. So if voyeurism is your bag (actually, a briefcase with a concealed camera in it is probably your bag) – check them out.

Watching your partner have sex or enjoy sexual intimacy with another person can be deeply traumatic – so even if you all get pissed and think it'll be a real laugh, it might not be the next morning. If you're bisexual it could work – on the basis that you get all the fun, and he hardly gets a look in. But what about the other woman? And what if he feels jealous? Because while 'two women' is the fantasy of most men, 'two women ignoring me' is not. The same goes for you – who wants to sit around watching her boyfriend getting off on someone else?

And if you decide it'd be a real laugh to take two men to bed, well, it might be as far as you're concerned. But unless your boyfriend is also bisexual it might simply spell complete jealousy and paranoia regarding sexual skills and penis-size.

So you see why it's fraught with danger. But, having said all that, if a threesome (or even sixsome) is what you've always wanted, and you're determined to try it, then there are ways of going about it that are less likely to end in total disaster. The 'total disaster' way involves one of you falling in love with the third party. So to avoid that, it may be better if you

> **TIP**
>
> If you want the thrills of a threesome without the risk towards your relationship, you can get a lot out of simply talking about it – describing what you'd do, and what the other man or woman would be doing to you both can be a turn-on too. Don't either of you however, discuss what his best mate, or your sister would be doing – that can be a little too much information for most. This way, you can enjoy your fantasy together without the danger. Cowards!

don't choose someone you're already intimate with – his best friend, for instance. Bad idea. And you don't want to spend the rest of your life wondering if your own best friend is still secretly fantasising about your partner's penis after one night of shared thrills. So to avoid all that (plus the ever-present danger of someone getting pissed and telling the packed local pub all about it) it's best to recruit a virtual stranger.

There used to be contact magazines for this sort of thing, and I always used to wonder how they did it once they'd made contact – 'Brian and Sheila? Ted and Angela. Lovely. Now, do have a few peanuts and a sherry, then we can get our clothes off and fuck.' I mean, really, how do you approach a complete stranger, or pair of strangers, and ask them if they'd like to have sex with you both? Luckily, the Internet has been a godsend for swingers. There are endless chat rooms where you can meet like-minded people, and check out their photographs before you sign up for an intimate session with a 15-stone trucker from Ohio. Should things go well, you'll exchange e-mails. And then, once you're all best buddies – which may take a couple of days – you'll arrange to meet up. How things progress from there is up to you, but it will probably involve some sort of offer of a 'massage'. If your third party is very upfront, though, he or she may simply shake hands and get naked. Well, it's what you wanted, isn't it?

You'll need to agree certain rules – whether that's 'no snogging the other people' or 'no intercourse with the others' or 'everything's allowed, but we don't discuss it afterwards …' Of course, I hardly need to tell you to use condoms. If you're advertising for sex on the net, chances are you're no virgin.

If you want to be more certain that you're getting a guy who isn't a total freak, however, you could try a male escort agency. That way, you'll have someone to complain to if he turns out to be a psychopath … just to look on the bright side for a moment.

If you're into proper swinging, as in visiting swingers' clubs and mingling with other naked swappers, you can usually find details in contact magazines. But be very sure of your reasons for getting into the scene – and if you're having sex with other couples, the rules are, if either of you feels remotely uncomfortable, you stop right away, however much fun your partner's having – and you never make assignations to see one of your

---

TIP

Take a leaf out of Sharon Stone's book – or at least, Sharon Stone as she was in *Sliver* and *Basic Instinct* – and go out without knickers, or else take them off while you're out and hand them to him as a little surprise present. Sharon did it, classily, under the table in the restaurant, which is always a good bet. If you bottle out, you can always nip to the loo and press them into his hot little hand. Knowing you're knickerless, even if he can't do anything about it, can lead to all sorts of filthy behaviour later. Unless he's called Nicholas, in which case it will just lead to silly jokes.

swappers behind your partner's back. Even if they have got a bigger penis. Actually, especially if they've got a bigger penis.

exhibitionism

Exhibitionism is basically just sexual showing-off. It's sex where you're being watched, or you could be discovered – sex with a real risk. Both partners have to find the idea exciting for exhibitionist sex to work, though if one's a voyeur, the exhibitionist can masturbate while he or she watches – some will even have sex with another person while their partner watches, but that's not terribly common. If both of you are show-offs though, it's a winner, as you'll both crave sex in supermarket car-parks, or to be filmed by the *Men and Motors* channel ...

Exhibitionism can be explored by taking pictures of each other – and sending them into the 'Readers' Wives and Husbands' sections of

---

TIP

If you decide to take a risk and go for sex outdoors, then choose your outfit with great care. In summer, it sounds dull, but covering yourself in insect repellent (then remembering not to lick it off) is also a useful precaution. Wear something long and floaty that you can drop to conceal yourself at a moment's notice, without knickers if possible. If you have to, a G-string is easier to push to one side than big knickers – and no bra is a must. He has less options than you, but trackies with an easily-adjusted elasticated waist are ultimately a lot more sensible than button-flies with a complex belt-buckle when it comes to speedy dressing.

> **TIP**
>
> Masturbating in public is a fantasy that a lot of people share – but actually doing it risks upsetting a great many passers-by and being done for indecent behaviour. So a device that does the stimulating for you, but no one knows, is probably the answer. You can get almost completely silent vibrators now, including one called The Whisperer – so, you're sitting on a boring train journey, you whip it out, pop it down your pants and off you go, with no one any the wiser. You could even try it in church – though I wouldn't recommend it. Duo balls are probably a better bet there.

porn mags. Then you can revel in how good you look next to the 45-year-old on the Dralon sofa with the tits like beanbags – and imagine everyone else getting off on your picture, too. Once again, our old friend the Internet plays a major part here – the world is the exhibitionist's oyster on the net. Webcams can record you undressing, masturbating, or having sex and beam it out to a grateful nation for less than the price of a weekend in Amsterdam. And if you're a voyeur – well, there are enough exhibitionists out there to satisfy your every desire. The only concern is safety – which you can ensure by never giving your personal details to anybody. And don't strip for the Webcam if the window behind you is right opposite Big Ben or anything – people can figure locations out surprisingly easily.

When it comes to having sex in public, swingers' clubs are the obvious port of call for the serious exhibitionist – no one's going to arrest you when half the guests are doing the same thing. If you get your jollies from giving him blow jobs in the middle of the shopping centre, however, you

If you really do feel like pushing the boat out exhibitionism-wise, you could do worse than try the popcorn wank, which takes place in the cinema. Wait till the lights go down – then, he gets his dick out, makes a hole in the bottom of the box, sticks it through, and guides your hand right on in there. You don't have much room to manoeuvre, but that's really beside the point – it's the sheer naughtiness that's a turn on. If you're nervous about being caught, though, go to an afternoon showing of a European art film, rather than the 8:00pm latest Tom Cruise. Just to be on the safe side.

need to be a little more careful, as it's entirely likely you'll be arrested. Consider (slightly) safer options such as sitting on his lap on a nightclub, wearing no knickers, and having sex that way, as clubbers dance around you. Just don't get carried away and let anything slip …

fetishism

A real fetish means you can't get aroused at all without your fetish-object. It's usually men who develop fetishes, and fixate their sexual feelings on a particular body part or object. Typical fetishes are shoes, feet, rubber, breasts – but they can go as far as car exhaust pipes, or even mud… For the purposes of adventurous sex, however, you're probably just playing around with the idea of a fetish – it's not that you can't manage without, it's just that adding something else arousing to the sexual mix provides a lovely *frisson* once in a while. Say for instance, high-heeled shoes, with ankle-ribbons. They elongate your legs, have a little hint of S&M about

> **TIP**
>
> If you are making a porn film, certain positions lend themselves to looking sexy on film – and guess what, it's not missionary. You leaning up against a wall, face-first, with your back arched so your arse sticks out looks great on film – and so does doggy-style, because to be blunt, it makes every woman's arse look fantastic. Typical porn poses show you off to best advantage, and allow the camera to pick up his penis going in and out – normal TV puts 10 pounds on, so maybe porn TV puts 10 inches on. There's always hope.

them, and most men find them hopelessly sexy. Or you could go for a transvestism fetish, and dress up as a man, while he dabs on make-up and puts on a dress. It may be a screamingly hilarious idea at first, but if he's a bit pretty, it can bring out whole other aspects of your personalities – whether dominant, submissive, feminine, masculine, you can really play around with roles in your sexual relationship.

Rubber, too, can be a highly sexy possibility – the true fetish often begins with the rubbery pants that children wear to protect their clothes

> **TIP**
>
> Keep the script short and to the point. Remember, the whole reason for making your porn film is to turn yourselves on watching it later. A load of waffle – 'my radiator's broken, can you fix it?' 'well, I don't know, I might need a spanner for that.' 'have you got one in the van?' 'I dunno, I'll go and look' – is not a sexy script. 'God, I want to have you now' is more effective when it comes to scripting.

from 'accidents' – sometimes men come to associate it with feelings of comfort and naughtiness. But even if the nearest you've ever got to rubber is a pencil eraser and your maths homework, the sensation of it on your skin can be arousing, as it's warm yet tight, and completely smooth. Rubber outfits can be very sexy – though if you're both rolling around in them, you'll be squeaking like a cageful of mice.

Fetishism can include black stockings, leather shorts (for him), full nurses' outfits, or even bandages. The good news is, when you both like it, you're both doing it in privacy, and so long as you're not nailing his penis to a plank of wood, with adventurous sex it really is a case of whatever (legally) turns you on …

7 advanced sex

Having advanced sex isn't actually that different from having un-advanced sex – it just means you'll do it more smoothly, your orgasms will be enhanced, and the whole thing will resemble the difference between drunkenly trying to dance the macarena by copying the person in front of you, and actually learning how to do it and understanding when you should jump in the air and put your hands on your shoulders. Ideally, though, the kind of sex you'll be having will provide you with slightly more fun than the macarena – unless you're a really, really good dancer, that is.

advanced kissing

I know we said right at the start that kissing is easy. It is, you really don't need to practice. But advanced kissing is slightly more complex. There are many different types of kiss – from 'Hi Gran' to the kind of nose-rub that means 'Brother Inuit, there is drifting snow on the tundra and the seals are dying,' to 'oh my god, my house, family and possessions are all going up in flames, but this feels so good, I just can't bring myself to care'. So to improve your own snogging repertoire, focus on the subtleties of kissing. Some believe there's a nerve that links the upper lip to the genitals – and who are you to prove them wrong? By nibbling on the lip, you can send messages of lust right through their body – so do it for a while, won't you? You can also indulge in butterfly kisses – typically, fluttering your eyelashes on his skin – but it can also mean tiny, featherlike kisses all over his face, finally concentrating on the corners of his mouth, and along his lips.

Then there's the Snake kiss – where you flick the tip of your tongue in and out, between his lips, and make brief contact with the tip of his tongue before pulling out again.

And the Soul kiss, where your tongues entwine, and you breathe into each other's mouths. Or even the kiss that is more of a suck – you suck on his lower lip, he sucks on your upper lip, and according to some *Kama Sutra*-toting sources, you can even have an orgasm this way. It may take a while though.

advanced foreplay
understanding each other's bodies

For good sex, it's essential that you understand how one another's bodies respond. When he touches your neck, you may experience an entirely different sensation from the one he feels when you touch his. And while you may love to have your nipples played with, for him it may just feel weird and mildly annoying. So it's worth devoting quite some time to practising different touches and caresses on different parts of each other. Techniques include stroking, biting, sucking, licking, pinching, and rubbing. Sex expert Anne Hooper calls this process 'body mapping'. She suggests that couples take turns to blindfold each other, and uses a scale of numbers to judge arousal – if they feel nothing, it's -3, if it's practically orgasmic, it's a +3 – a very handy way for your partner to know what's worth bothering with, and what isn't. Focus on one small area at a time, and concentrate fully on the sensations you're feeling.

If his penis errs on the side of small, then a handy tip is to wait until it's really big before you let him enter you – and the best way to maximise penis-potential is by sucking it, hard. Once you really don't believe it can get any bigger without a vacuum pump, roll a ribbed condom over it – this will create the friction that may be lacking from a really small one. And if you also adopt one of the 'deep entry' positions – which you'll know if you've been paying attention – you'll barely know the difference between him and a normal-sized guy. Don't mention that, obviously.

stroking

Stroking is perfect for a general relaxation session. He should stroke you by alternating small, brushing motions and big, sweeping motions, all over. Your back, bum, thighs – both inner and outer – and arms will probably respond well to stroking. When it's his turn, focus on the sides of his torso – a highly neglected area – inner thighs and his bum. Many men are less sensitive in their limbs than women are, so don't waste endless time trailing your fingers up and down his calves, it's probably not worth your while.

biting

If you use it carefully, biting can be intensely erotic. Make sure you take your cue from your partner when it comes to how hard to clamp your teeth together, though – an arousing nip is not the same thing as a blood-drawing chew. Good places for biting on you are your neck, just below your ears and at the back – gently – your earlobes, buttocks, inner thighs, and your sides. Biting breasts is rarely a good plan, unless he does it as if he was holding a little baby fairy between his teeth. And even then, go easy. On him, earlobes, inner thighs, neck, bum, sides – all can benefit from light biting.

sucking

The main focus of attention here is almost certainly going to be breasts. He should suck gently, though, not as if he's trying to unblock a sink. And he can also try it on your thighs, fingers (very erotic), earlobes, and – if he's inclined to – toes. You should suck his – well, obviously his willy, but it's hardly news that that feels good, is it? – fingers (because it reminds him of having his willy sucked), earlobes, balls, and – are you sure you want to do this? – toes. Maybe.

licking

Licking is good news as far as your neck, ears, collarbone, breasts, bum, back, and thighs are concerned. In fact, there are few places that don't benefit from a nice little lick. He should run his tongue down your spine, flicker it into the crevice at the top of your buttocks, and circle the tip lovingly on your inner thighs. You, meanwhile, should focus your licking efforts on his neck, ears, nipples, hips, bum, balls and inner thighs. That's a lot of tongue-work …

pinching

Pinching can be oddly arousing – if it's done lightly, and in the right places. It's good for your bum, nipples, and inner thighs – on him, the same is probably true. Pinching anywhere else just looks like cruelty – and don't even think about trying it with his penis, will you?

rubbing

Some people are so sensitive that if you rub them too hard in one spot, they'll develop a sore patch – which is, really, not what you want at all. But a little gentle rubbing can work wonders on necks, inner elbows, back of knees, spines – and here is where feet come into their own, because while you may not want to bite, nibble or suck them, almost everyone loves having their feet rubbed.

By understanding exactly what works when it comes to touching each other, you'll ensure that you don't waste hours poking and prodding in completely the wrong places, wondering why you aren't getting the response you hoped for. What's more, your foreplay will be streamlined so perfectly that your partner may well be trembling on the verge of an orgasm before you even reach their genitals. Which is a good thing.

advanced orgasm

Right, sit up and pay attention. Advanced orgasm is not as difficult as it sounds. But it turns out there are different types, and according to Lou Paget, men can experience an orgasm in up to seven different ways, and women in up to ten different ways. Now, don't feel insecure about this, it's merely to give you an inkling of the possibilities, nobody's suggesting you should be having ten different kinds of orgasm or else you're not enjoying yourself – fun's fun, and if it feels good, just one kind's fine by most of us. But just so you know, the ways men can experience orgasm are, apparently, via intercourse, manual, oral, prostate, fantasy/dreams, touching or sucking breasts, and sex toys. Doesn't sound that complicated now, does it? Although most men past the age of 14 might have trouble coming from

> **TIP**
>
> The two-handed hand job is a winner, because it ensures your clit feels great, without putting any excess pressure on it – this one works very well if you've had a lot of stimulation lately (I know, you should be so lucky) and your clitoris can't take any direct action. He just needs to place one hand over the other, then put both of them over your pubic mound, and rub slowly. The spreading of pressure across a wider area means that you'll get new, thrilling sensations, but you won't orgasm for a while, which may suit you very well.

just breast contact alone. As for women, they can orgasm via clitoral, vaginal and cervical (no I don't know what the big difference is there, either) stimulation, G-spot, urethra, breast contact, mouth contact, anal, blended/fusion, zone and fantasy.

Alright, now we really are in the realms of sci-fi. It's just about acceptable that certain very specific individual women may possibly be able to come through merely being kissed. We suspect, however, that these women are lonely nuns, suddenly surprised by manly motorcyclists, who have roared into the convent grounds and crushed the startled sisters against their manly, leather-clad chests … hang on, I'm beginning to understand … fair enough. But Blended and Fusion? Zone? Are these orgasms or diets, for heaven's sake?

In truth, it's relatively simple. Ish. A Blended or Fusion orgasm means that more than one area of the body is being stimulated. I bet you never knew that him playing with your nipple and your clitoris simultaneously had a special, grown-up name, did you? Well, now you do. A Zone orgasm, meanwhile (oh, do keep up!) just means you've orgasmed from having an area of the body stimulated that wouldn't normally lead to an orgasm. So if he's rubbing your nose and suddenly you're overcome with waves of pulsating sensation, you'll know you've had a Zone orgasm. Or possibly you've sneezed.

his and hers

It should be becoming clear by now that men and women have markedly different experiences of orgasm. Which is why simultaneous orgasm is so rare. Forget all the films you've ever seen where they're at it like ferrets in a bag, then suddenly they both go all eye-rolling and start shouting 'uh! Yes! Oh god!' and collapse in a heap at the same time. She's so faking it. Well, so is he, he's acting, but if they were real people she would be, too. Because simultaneous orgasm hardly ever happens through penetration, though it can occasionally occur through mutual masturbation, so long as you speed it up and then slow it down, as Bucks Fizz once famously sang, to match your partners' rate of arousal. Which makes sex sound about as exciting as test-driving a Fiat Uno, but still. And if he is still bleating on about why you aren't having multiple, award-winning orgasms during sex, you may wish to point out that 28% of women can't come at all during sex, with or without clitoral stimulation. Though I couldn't begin to imagine how they found that out – 'excuse me, Madame, we're conducting a survey ...'

Anyhow, the joy of simultaneous orgasm is a myth. Because even if you do manage to achieve one, you're both so busy galloping along your own little race-tracks to the finishing line, you don't pay any attention to each other – and surely at least part of the point of sex is to enjoy your partner's responses?

The best way to do it, if possible, is for you to come first, and then let him come. Otherwise, he'll come, then go all comatose and sleepy because he's been flooded with dopamine, and you'll be left to finish the job your-self, whether you like it or not. Oh, he'll make some half-hearted hand-flap-ping attempt, but if you want to be sure of decent orgasms all round, try to get yours in first.

advanced anatomy

It's not that you need a degree in advanced human biology to enjoy sex or anything – but it's nice to be able to pinpoint the important bits of your inner workings, should the need arise. So with that in mind, here's a quick refresher course on where to find all those spots ... let's call it the Dalmatian Course.

g-spot

You'll find this around 2 inches up on the front inner wall of the vagina. It's an area of soft, ridgy or spongy tissue, the size of a penny, but it swells to ... ooh, at least a 10p ... when correctly stimulated. If you're looking for it (and hey, aren't we all, honey?) you need to squat on all fours right after stimulation, so it's engorged and easier to locate – then get your fingers right up there and wiggle them around. Or he can.

a-spot

It's further up than the G-spot, another spongy little spot, on the front inner wall again. To find it – you may need a dildo or extra-long, pianist's fingers for this – use a light pressing motion on the front wall, and push down with your abdominal muscles to heighten the sensations. Leaning backwards may help – but if you can't find it, you're in good company.

When searching for the G-spot, it helps if you go for a wee first – otherwise, all that prodding about near the bladder can prove highly distracting, as it puts pressure on the sphincter muscles, and suddenly you'll need the loo just as things are getting good. Some women like the sensation of a full bladder and find it increases their chances of orgasm – but if you're not one of them, make sure you go before you go, as your gran used to say. Though she probably didn't mean it like that.

c-spot

This is the spot right at the neck of your cervix – and you need to go very carefully here, because banging around up there can hurt. After all, smear tests aren't the biggest laugh going, are they? But if you get it right, you can experience deep and giddy sensations from the C-spot. Getting it right, however, takes effort. Try hooking your ankles over his shoulders and raising your bum so you're tipped backwards – that's about as deep as penetration gets, and you stand a fair chance of bumping it – but tell him to go gently. Easier is an extra-long vibrator with a rounded tip, which may well stimulate the spot in question through gentle buzzing.

u-spot

It's surrounded on three sides by the clitoris and its environs, so stimulation here is sure to result in some kind of excitement, even if it does make you want to wee. He can locate this one for you, in a most pleasant fashion, by placing his lower lips over his teeth during oral sex (yes, he'll look like a gurning granddad, but who cares?) and applying light pressure on the spot in question. And it will respond remarkably well to a soft, gentle tongue stroke.

female ejaculation

We all know about male ejaculation. It's called semen, it contains sperm, it looks like ectoplasm, and it goes everywhere when you give hand jobs. Simple. Female ejaculation, however, is a whole different ballgame. There is controversy as to whether it actually exists – some think it's wee, but there is definitely a colourless fluid that can be ejaculated from the vagina at the point of orgasm. It may simply be lubrication that's collected in a pool, and a muscle spasm shoots it out at once ... who knows, it may be pixies' special lemonade, whatever, but if you want to try it, you need to be aroused to the point of orgasm, then as you feel the first contraction, bear down hard with your abdominal muscles, as though you're trying to shoot peas off your stomach. It may or may not happen – but there's no harm in trying.

TIP

When giving him a blow job, twist your tongue around the tip every time you come up the shaft. You don't need to be too rhythmic – just alternate between clockwise and anti-clockwise, or swirl it around as if you're licking a cornet packed with delicious ice-cream. The contrast between your sucking action and the little extra swirling sensation on the most sensitive area should make him forget why penises were invented in the first place – he'll believe it was simply for this.

If you want to swallow when you give him a blow job, certain foods make his semen taste much nicer – and the best thing he can drink to improve the flavour is pineapple juice. Maybe give him some coconut milk too, then you'll get the whole pina colada thing going on … but the enzymes in pineapple juice have a sweetening effect on his secretions, so force it down him. Foods he should avoid include tobacco, caffeine, and asparagus. You can also try going down on him with a swig of mild mouthwash – it's exciting for him, and masks the taste of any asparagus-based semen for you.

advanced oral sex

Oral sex? Come on, surely you know it all by now! But wait, there's still a little information that may be to your advantage …

69

69 position … been there, done that? You sure? OK, but did you enjoy it? That's the trouble with 69, it really is way too much like rubbing your tummy and patting your head. It's far too complicated to get comfortable enough to enjoy a proper, relaxed orgasm – you're too busy trying to avoid getting cramp in your neck, or your jaw seizing up, and he's struggling to breathe. But that's the classic 69 position, where you lie with your bodies alongside each other, you've got your head stuffed between his legs, he's got his stuffed between yours, and that's not accounting for the fact that both your bodies are jack-knifed uncomfortably, due to the height difference between you.

This is not the best way to get the most out of it. What you should be doing is this: you lie on your back, and he crouches above you, facing your feet. That way you get to give him a blow job and play with his balls, which are miraculously accessible, and he gets to go down on you upside down, which is highly enjoyable, and means he can also reach a finger into your vagina.

You can do the position in reverse – you crouching over him – but that involves slightly more work for you, which is obviously less desirable.

blow job

For the ultimate blow job, it works best if you're crouching between his legs while he sits on the edge of the bed, or a chair. He can stand and lean against a wall, if he prefers. Being on your knees may be a little subservient but it gives you a lot more room for manoeuvre. That way, too, he can look down and see exactly what your tongue is doing. With one hand, reach underneath to caress his balls, and form your mouth into a hard 'o' for the best sensation you can offer. If your lips are too floppy you could be there for hours, getting a numb jaw. The best way to bring matters to a swift con-

---

TIP

Men can actually strengthen their tongues in the same way they can practice to strengthen their PC muscles. A particularly useful exercise to get his tongue used to moving in a different way from its usual pattern of tasting chips and beer and talking, is for him to lick out a pot of yoghurt – or crème fraiche if he's posh. The necessity of extracting every last drop will mean he has to extend his tongue like a python, and rotate it gently – which is excellent practise when he comes to do the same for your own, er, yoghurt pot …

> **TIP**
>
> If he's going down on you, it's vital he shaves first – unless he has enough stubble-growth to make it soft. If he does, pressing his chin lightly against your vagina will create a series of prickles that feels fantastic as he moves his face. Which he should do – far too many men seem to think they have to assume one head-position and use their tongue to do all the work, whereas actually moving his head around allows him much greater access to all your nooks and crannies. Hence the need not to have agonisingly painful stubble.

clusion is with strong, powerful sucking action- – it may be a little harsh on the cheeks but he'll appreciate it so much it's almost worth it. Move your head back and forth, and meantime, flicker your tongue across the tip of his penis, and up and down, quickly and lightly. When he starts to make 'about to come' noises, don't stop – this is not the time to pull away and say 'are you about to come in my mouth?' Just keep on truckin' and – yes – let him come in your mouth, swallow, and even try and pretend you enjoyed it. Easy.

cunnilingus

The ultimate is simply getting it right, which is harder than it sounds. But to give you the best blow job you've ever had, he needs to bear a few things in mind. Lying right between your legs is out – but lying with his head at right angles, so it's pillowed on your thigh and his fingers can reach in to spread your labia, is definitely in. To make it easier for him, you can raise your other leg to give him more access. He should begin with the Kivin method (see previous chapter for details) before moving on to stimulate the U-spot with soft gentle licks. Circling movements are required, and he shouldn't take his tongue away. At the same time, he can insert a finger in your vagina to press on the G-spot, and press another against your anus. He can, if he has the coordination of a Russian ice-dancer, reach his other hand up and play with your breasts and nipples. As long as he remembers the watchwords 'light' and 'gentle' it can only be a matter of minutes before a shattering orgasm overtakes you.

'hovering butterfly'

'Sit on my face' is generally used as more of a crude insult than a romantic invitation – however, if we cunningly change the description to Lou Paget's far more sensitive 'hovering butterfly,' the experience becomes instantly more attractive. Sitting on his face is more a matter of suspending yourself above his face – if you actually sat on it, he'd suffocate, which may be an admirable way to go, but is perhaps a little unnecessarily dramatic. The best way to do it is by holding onto something behind his head – like the bed-head – otherwise your thigh muscles will go into spasm halfway through. If there's nothing to hold onto, lean forward, and put your hands on the wall. The beauty of this position is that he has full access both visually and phys-ically – he can part your labia with his fingers, and see exactly what he's doing and where, with his tongue. He can also reach your breasts and bum – so if you can overcome your inhibitions, face-sitting is a great way to enjoy advanced oral sex. Note, however, that him sitting on your face really does-n't work – unless you have a whole anal thing going on.

advanced anal

Talking of whole anal things, advanced play in this area can result in some stunning orgasms and sensations. And it's not the once-in-a-lifetime exper-

TIP

For you, anal sex can be made infinitely more appealing if you're pre-pared to let him lick your anus. If Charlotte in *Sex & the City* can do it, you can too. As long as you're squeaky-clean it's harmless, and because the anus is rich in nerve-endings, it can feel thoroughly delightful to have him run his tongue around it. This is known as 'rimming,' but 'rosebudding,' it's other name, is a little prettier. He can put his tongue inside your anus, but it's not advisable, due to free-floating bacteria. If you're keen, purchase a Dental Dam – very paranoid-American, but very safe.

iment it used to be – a Playboy survey reveals that 47% of men and 67% of women have tried anal intercourse … which begs the question, who or what were the extra 20% of women having it with? Looks like somebody's lying … or else they're lesbians, and counting penetration with dildos as intercourse, or there's a few men out there having anal sex with lots of dif-ferent women. Let's hope they're using condoms. Interestingly, the biggest increase in sex toys is in anal toy sales, so if everybody's at it, surely it pays to know exactly what's worth bothering with.

For him, anal penetration will usually be with fingers. You need to

TIP

You can buy a butt plug – a charmingly romantic name, I'm sure you'll agree – which inserts into the anus. Some actually vibrate, and the inflating sort expands to twice its original size, in order to stim-ulate the male G-spot.

insert a very well-lubricated finger about an inch and a half, to a point where you'll feel two sphincter muscles against the side when you press – the gland you're looking for is another couple of inches in, on the front wall, and when touched feels sensational.

how to delay male orgasm

As at least half this book is dedicated to the pursuit of orgasm, it seems a little strange to be attempting to put it off. But some men – though not many women – do suffer from the curse of premature ejaculation, which means that nobody's getting quite as much fun as they could be having. There are, however, ways of avoiding this – chief amongst which is the stop-start technique.

He enters you, and thrusts to the point just before orgasm is inevitable. Then he pulls out, waits for the feelings to subside for a few seconds – he can continue to touch you while he waits, though – and then

---

TIP

One simply lovely tip to hold back male orgasm is for him to imagine he's going for a pooh and activate the same muscles (but not that much that he really … oh god, oh god, stop there). This has the interesting effect of preventing orgasm, in much the same way as images of nuns, or grannies in big knickers, are alleged to. For you, however, if you want to encourage orgasm, the best thing you can do with your muscles is to clench your lower stomach hard, as your excitement begins to peak. This can intensify and prolong your orgasm – if you just forget the fact that he's thinking about pooh.

---

re-enters you, carries on again, till he feels orgasm approaching like a runaway train, then pulls out again … This can continue until you're both satisfied, at which point he's finally allowed to come.

Another method, if you can't be bothered with all the stopping and starting, or if he doesn't have a problem with it, you just want to go on longer, is the Squeeze technique. Just before he comes, make a ring around the base of his penis with your thumb and forefinger and squeeze lightly. This should stop the semen that thinks it's on its way to victory, and buy you a little more time. But really, don't squeeze too hard. That's just mean.

advanced sex toys

As was seen in Chapter 5, the world of sex toys has many places to explore – and new ones are constantly being designed. Ultimately, they're all there to ensure your orgasm – but the routes they offer to get you there are increasingly fascinating. Toys specially designed for anal sex, which feature a flange to stop it lodging in your rectum, are available – not to mention the 'Wee Willie,' with a slim, angled shaft and a rounded shaft which you can either wear in a harness or use manually … I'd love to have been at the marketing meeting for these things. You can also get a vibrating 'tail spin,' a dildo that offers a tail that spins gently inside your anus. It sounds a little too much like some kind of weird bottom-toothbrush to be truly sensual, but it may be worth a go.

For vaginal/clitoral excitement, however, you may want to invest in a vibrating love-cushion, which does exactly what it says – you switch it on, sit on it, and before you know it, you're having wild orgasms with no hands involved. It feels kind of like when the bus stops and the engine's still on, only better. And without the school kids throwing bags around.

The Tongue Joy, meanwhile, is a vibrating bullet-shaped attachment that fixes to your tongue with a little strap, and allows anywhere you lick to also be vibrated. It may feel weird for the user, but it feels damn hot for the one experiencing it. Just don't swallow it in your excitement.

There's also The Octopus. It fits round the penis, with clit-stimulator attached (though why they didn't call it the Octopussy is a mystery to me) and the flexible vibrator, which can reach pretty much any spot – G, C, U, or A – you like. Hell, you can even get the Pony-Play butt plug, a cute little device with a horse's tail that makes you look like a real pony … but I suspect that's a little too advanced, even for me.

advanced thrusting

Thrusting isn't that difficult – all he has to do is plunge in and out, aided by your hip movements, in a bid to create friction. Anyone can, and does, do it. Advanced thrusting, however, relies on maintaining a certain level of control. He needs to build up his PC muscle, by hanging a flannel on his penis and raising and lowering it – look, good sex takes work, you know.

But by learning to control his speed and power of thrust, he can improve the sexual experience for both of you. Try it with several short thrusts, followed by one sudden, deep thrust – the more unexpected, the better it is for you, but don't try it in a deep-penetration position, it's best in missionary.

You can also train your PC muscles to the extent that you can have sex without moving, once he's inside you. You sitting on top is the best position by far for this. He inserts his penis inside you, and you squeeze it with your vagina, in a series of short contractions. The stronger the muscles, the better it will feel for him – if they're gladiator-strength, you can make him come this way, but it takes a lot of practice. He'll thank you for it, though.

You can also enjoy slower, more erotic sex by rotating your hips together, rather than actually thrusting – this has the added effect of grinding on your clitoris, and stimulating the full area of your vaginal wall.

advanced roleplay

With fantasy, as stated in Chapter 4, the only thing to bear in mind is whether your partner actually wants to know or not. If not, you're somewhat hampered when it comes to acting it out. If so, however, there's little to stop you except the fear that it won't be as good in real life. The truth is, you're right, it might not be. But one fantasy nearly always works as a role-play – the Strangers in the Night fantasy. Having sex with a stranger is one of the top fantasies enjoyed by both men and women. Although he or she may be faceless – and fantasy lovers often are – it's the knowledge that you won't be judged, nobody will know, and that you can be completely uninhibited that gives the imaginary encounter its excitement, unhampered by relationship issues, insecurities, and real life. It's a simple transaction of desire and being desired in its most basic form. Now, if you were to enact this in real life, your partner would, understandably, be thoroughly annoyed, and may well leave you. As a shared fantasy, however, it's perfectly possible to act it out, highly convincingly.

You need to arrange – via text message, if possible, to make it detached – to both be in a hotel bar at a certain time. You must arrive separately – it's no use setting out together. He arrives first, books a room, and settles down in the bar in the manner of a jaded business traveller. You get all dressed up, shave your legs, wax your pubic hair (unless that gives you a nasty rash) and generally prepare to go out on the pull. Then, you turn up in the bar, and take a separate table. After a while, he sends a drink over to your table. You smile in acknowledgement … and after a while, you invite him over. You talk about anything but your personal lives – and you don't ever crack a smile of complicity, or let on that this is a game – you'll ruin it. Saying 'just a minute, did you hang the washing out before you left?' will be the end of everything.

After a while, you start flirting big-time. Others in the bar will watch as you fondle his knee, and he strokes your arm. And they will watch open-mouthed as you head for the lifts together, then proceed to the room he's booked and have mind-blowing sex. Afterwards, you may want to end the game. Or you may want to carry on, leave, return to him, and greet him the next day without ever mentioning your night of illicit passion in the arms of a stranger.

advanced behaviour

Sexual behaviour that's not advanced is no longer part of your repertoire, of course. But there's just a couple more things that need mentioning. Like, initiating sex. Far too many couples rely on the man to do all the initiation – then they wonder why they fall into a pattern where he's pestering, and she's tutting and moaning about being tired. If you make a conscious effort, however, to initiate it yourself – and you'd be depressed to learn how few long-term couples actually bother to snog more than once every few weeks – you'll be amazed at how much it perks up your sex life. He'll feel wanted, you'll feel sensual and uninhibited, and those feelings will miracu-lously translate into your sex life.

8 spiritual sex

Spiritual sex is the kind you don't have with a one-night stand. While it can be passionate, its whole point is about forging a deeper connection between you. Staring into each other's eyes is par for the course, but you'll also be expected to breathe into each other's mouths, and generally unite in a bubble of one-ness on the path to orgasm. The reward for all this intimacy and patience is, of course, the greatest orgasm known to man – the full body orgasm, or FBO as those in the know like to call it.

Along the way, though, you should grow in your spiritual understanding of each other – and ideally, learn how not to feel silly whilst pulling a penis to unleash the Chi energy. Actually, that might be something you have to come to terms with yourself.

Some of the moves are a direct descendant from yoga – and others are connected to the Eastern philosophies and their belief in Chi energy points, or chakras. Basically, this is not the sexual technique you'll want for a quickie.

connecting with your sexual energy

Non-tantric sex has a beginning, middle and end – it's a very linear process, which goes from arousal to plateau to orgasm, and it can take less than 15 minutes. In fact, as we all know, occasionally it can take less than 5. And given that a lot of women need a good 20 minutes (or even a very average 20 minutes) to reach full arousal, that can't be good.

Tantric sex, by contrast, is approached as circular activity – there's no designated final credits where 'The End' rolls in loopy writing over a scene of the two of you sharing a cigarette. The 'being in the moment of union' is what it's all about – experiencing every sensation fully, without leaping ahead to the end as fast as possible. The good part is, it's not all just look-into-my eyes stuff – it also regularly features several orgasms in a single session. No wonder Sting always looks so relaxed.

For spiritual sex, you need to build up your sexual energies by slowing the process right down. In your case, you can begin to prepare by slowly massaging your breasts – start at the edges and work inwards, in small, slow circles. This apparently keeps your mind focused on the sex

---

TIP

A Taoist exercise called the Golden Circle can help you to direct sexual energy from the pelvic area through the rest of the body. Sit with your eyes closed and relax your tongue so it sits just behind your teeth, then focus your attention on your pelvic girdle – it's the bones of your hips, pubic area and lower back, and it's bowl-shaped. Visualise it filled with warm golden honey, then imagine it flowing in a tube from your spine to the top of your head. When it reaches the top, hold your breath for five seconds, then breathe out as it flows back down. Hold it for a minute as it reaches the bowl again. Don't strain – just stop for a moment if it's not happening for you. The idea is to move Chi through your body, and your imagination can help its flow.

> **TIP**
>
> Your skin is your biggest erogenous zone, and breast skin is particularly thin and therefore sensitive – so he shouldn't ignore its potential. Going straight for the nipples means missing out on a whole world of stimulation, when he should be swirling his fingertips across the skin of your breasts, and tracing them along the underside to awaken a whole bunch of nerves you never even knew were there. Stroking, however, is not the same thing as squashing – so make sure he doesn't start treating them like plasticine.

organs – but a handy knock-on effect is that it also encourages the flow of blood to your breasts and makes them increase in size. It's called Chi massage, and the male version requires him to rub his perineum, and massage his testicles with two fingers, using a light, gentle stroke, for several minutes.

He should then grasp the end of his penis – not an instruction that many men resent – whilst breathing out, and bend over, pushing his tongue out and pulling on his penis. Yes, indeed it looks hilariously stupid. But if it builds up sexual energy, then who are you to argue with the ancient Taoists? The exercises aren't done with the aim of viewing intercourse as the goal – it's merely a staging post along the way to Nirvana, alright?

And there are certain things you need to do before you even think about having sex that will ensure that when you do, it's a thing of beauty and a joy forever.

The first stage is to find out what turns your partner on – without expecting that the discussion will turn into sex. You're expected to make your relationship a priority – even if you have kids, or highly demanding careers, and can't spare the time that would have been available to a courtesan of

> **TIP**
>
> Women prefer wildly differing strengths of nipple-suction – so to make sure that he isn't treating them like he's trying to get an extra-thick milkshake through a cocktail straw, just suck on his tongue to show him what you'd like him to do. You could suck on his nipples, but they're less sensitive than yours, whereas his tongue is highly sensitive – unless he's a heavy smoker who exists on extra-strong curries … in which case you probably don't want to be going anywhere near his mouth.

an ancient Emperor, you can still set aside at least an hour or two a week to devote to yourselves, without the TV or the children blaring in the background. You will also be expected to make the atmosphere reasonably pleasant – so rendezvousing in a bedroom overflowing with laundry and old newspapers will do bad things, feng shui wise. You may not be able to turn it into the required 'sacred space' with five minutes and only a bin bag at your disposal, but you can certainly light some candles, and stick a few flowers in a vase. Scented candles are ideal, as the relaxing, or sensual ones, will put you in the mood much faster than the smell of next door's curry. At the very least, switch a lamp on, instead of that glaring overhead 60-watt thing, and play some suitable music – something like *Buddha Bar*, Claude Challe's orient-inspired mixes, should do the job – or a little Mozart if that's your bag. Not Marilyn Manson, though.

Pay attention to what you wear, too – knackered jogging bottoms aren't perhaps the most sensual of outfits for either of you. Or have baths or showers first – a good plan anyway – and turn up in the manner of Marilyn Monroe, wearing nothing but Chanel No. 5. He will, of course, be wearing aftershave. Accessorise yourself with jewellery, long, seductive ear-rings or necklaces – go easy on the rings, though, you don't want to do him a nasty mischief.

intimacy

Ritual is used in tantra to develop intimacy – not your normal ritual, how-ever, of 'where's the remote?', 'you're sitting on it', 'do you want a cup of tea?' – but a far more seductive one. At least, we can only hope so.

Food is a good basis for ritual – and finger food is even better, because you can feed each other. Obviously, we're not talking about Scotch eggs, or sausage rolls, but seductive food like fruit, asparagus (though it does make your wee smell terrible) and chocolates. Wine is also a good bet at this point, to overcome any lingering inhibitions, plus it's been used in rituals of one sort or another since time immemorial. Or your ritual could be as simple as bathing together, in lovely scented water.

As long as you're focusing on each other positively, whether that takes the form of a game of cards or a prolonged poetry-reading session, you're on the right track.

If you're really keen to go with the whole idea of tantric sex, you'll be doing this for some weeks before you consider moving onto sex – it's all about building up the anticipation, though you may feel that's pushing things a bit far. Hey, I'm only telling you what some people do …

breathing control

Do you ever think about breathing? It's unlikely, it being simply a matter of processing enough air in and out to stay alive. But in tantric sex, breathing matters, trust me. Shared breathing, however, is a power-ful way to bring you closer, and help you focus on each other. Sit facing each other cross-legged, like you did at Playgroup. Put your hands on your knees, palms up, and look into your partner's eyes, taking slow, deep breaths. You may feel like a prize prat, but it's worth keeping on, honest.

Breathe at the same rate, in through your nose and out through your mouth (you can chant 'in with anger, out with love' at the same time if you want to, but possibly not). Ideally, you'll be able to maintain this breathing, coupled with eye contact, for a good 10 minutes or so. Then and only then are you allowed to touch each other. It's alleged that some couples achieve orgasm through 'soul gazing' alone. I'm sure they have, and I'd love to meet them.

erotic touch

You are now allowed to touch – hurrah! But it's back to Anne Hooper's body mapping, not wild sex – you're just touching each other gently, and talking about what feels good. Tell each other where you want to be stroked or caressed, whether you'd prefer it to be with fingers or tongue, and be appreciative when each other gets it right.

According to tantric teaching, the longer you build up sexual energy, the longer men can avoid orgasming. Start your actual love-making session by kissing each other all over – it's important that you don't start breath-ing heavily, like a marathon runner, as soon as the excitement kicks in. Panting hurries you towards orgasm, but deep, slow, measured breaths will hold it off. If you now start breathing alternately – he breathes out as you breathe in – you'll be more connected.

If you are breathing into each other's mouths though, be careful – you don't want to build up so much carbon dioxide you go all faint and dizzy. At least, not for any reason other than lust.

positions

In tantra, different positions are used to increase pleasure as well as balancing Chi energy. So men are expected to take female 'subservient' roles as well as the more traditional dominant ones, which frees them to engage on a more emotional level, while you can be more direct and demanding than is traditionally expected. Of course, nowadays, that's not so unusual, but come on – at the time it was wild. So you might adopt the traditional missionary, but with the positions reversed, so you're leaning over him, or he might be the inner 'spoon' that fits to your body while you caress his penis.

All that Flaying of the Goat *Kama Sutra* stuff is not strictly necessary – I mean, you can if you want, but tantra isn't about bending your legs behind your ears, it's just about making a connection.

TIP

If his penis is bigger than your vaginal opening, it may cause problems. Don't be alarmed – it can stretch – but it's vital that you allow lots of time for foreplay. One useful way to handle it, though, is for you to come before he tries to penetrate you – a relaxed vagina makes an enormous difference to how easy it is to get inside, so by ensuring you're fully wet and relaxed, it'll be a lot less painful when he tries. He must go slowly though, and the best position is woman on top, so you can control the speed and depth of thrusting.

multiple for men

Orgasm and ejaculation are separate in tantra-world, and we already know that he can come without actually ejaculating. But the exciting bit is, rather than just showing off and allowing his sperm to end up lying around in his bladder instead of on the sheet, by doing this he can experience a series of mini-orgasms, within a controlled climax. According to tantra, he is simply surfing the energy wave, without drowning in it. To do so, he can put various tricks – I mean, modes of tantric enlightenment – into practice. He can clench the PC muscles, as explained in Chapter 3, in a series of short bursts. He can also consciously relax – as soon as he feels his orgasm overtaking him, he should take a deep breath, and pause in his thrusting – similar to the stop-start technique. Don't let his erection collapse altogether, though.

If he tightens his PC muscles every time his arousal peaks, it should hold off orgasm for quite some time. In fact, you could still be there next Tuesday, wondering when he'll finally get around to it. To have his flow of mini-orgasms, he needs to finally clench his PCs and take a deep breath at the same time – it's hard to pick the exact moment, though, so don't be surprised if it all goes pear- (or ectoplasm-) shaped a few times first. When he gets it, though, he'll be ecstatic … and you'll be … well, concentrating on your own orgasm, presumably.

your tantric orgasm

Obviously, clitoral stimulation is expected – nay, demanded. But the old G-spot rears its spongy head again here, because in tantra it's known as the Sacred Spot. So yes, once again you'll be unfolding the map and hoping for the best – only this time, it's spiritual. A good grasp of tantra should mean that you can direct energy through the body's chakras, which builds up sensations of heightened pleasure.

ways of touching

Tantric touching is the key to all pleasure (oh, apart from breathing) and it's important that you change the style of your touching every minute or so – except during oral sex, that is, in which case the rule is, if it ain't broke, don't fix it. Alternating touch, however, builds up sexual energy. It's useful to look for areas of each other's bodies that feel cool, then caress them till they warm up – that way you release even more energy. In fact, you're releasing so much by now you could probably bottle it and sell it as Tantric Viagra.

where to begin

Start your touching with each other's faces, where the nose meridian is connected to the root chakra. Extend your stroking downwards, through each other's necks, arms, breasts/torso, stomach, genitals, and then go back, completing the body-circle of touching – even if he's begging you to stick with the genitals. By doing this, you're creating an energy circuit. See, it's just like physics.

TIP

Chakras are energy centres in the body. The 'root chakra' is sexual energy that resides at the base of the spine, near the anus. So don't ignore it.

For you, he should gently suck and lick your upper lip, so his lower lip rubs against the connecting tissue between your gums and upper lips – this apparently has a direct line to the clitoris. You may not orgasm from this alone, but there's no harm trying, is there?

For him, stimulate the area where his shoulders join his neck. This part responds very well to biting and nibbling, and even sucking. You need to move up the back of the neck to the base of the skull – doing this releases pent-up tension, and this area lies on meridians, or energy channels, that connect to his pelvis.

You can gain pleasure from having the thyroid glands, located on either side of your throat just under the earlobe, stimulated – all he needs to do is slowly stroke them with his fingertips to turn you on even more, then run his hands down onto your breasts and nipples, which, of course, have a direct hotline to your clitoris.

More esoterically, if he caresses your wrist bones, this simple act can drive you wild, and also, apparently, it will transmit energy to the heart, and increase your emotional passion.

Another good spot for both of you to caress is the 'elixir field' (really!), which is the area just above her pubic bone that's very rich in nerve-endings. You can both just place your hands there, and let the energies course through your bodies – in your case, this should stimulate the G-spot externally, and focus your sensations on the area, whereas in his, it's close to his willy, so it just feels nice.

Now it gets good. You can experience a labial massage – what one sexpert calls 'wibbling'. He should simply massage your outer labia – without opening it, or entering. He can also caress the inner thighs, creating a circle of stroking. With his fingertips he can 'wibble' the soft skin of your labia, by pinching it lightly between finger and thumb, but he mustn't touch

---

TIP

In the early stages of penetration, shallow thrusting is better because it directly stimulates the areas of your vagina that are most sensitive to pressure. When the head of his penis moves back and forth, this builds up your excitement. It also means that when he goes in more deeply, the upper areas are more ready to respond, because you've built up desire. Shallow thrusting also encourages your vagina to contract, in an attempt to keep him inside you, which is exciting for him too. If he then penetrates you deeply, pulls out again, and thrusts shallowly, it creates a vacuum that tugs at the vaginal walls. And guess how good that feels?

---

your clitoris. I hardly need tell you that this feels nice. And the bonus is, it moves energy around your pelvis too – you can't lose.

One technique used by Taoists is the '5-minute' technique, whereby you take turns to stimulate each other in whatever ways possible, for 5 minutes each. After that, you must swap over – however desperate you are to continue. If you want built-up sexual energy ... well, there's your method.

full body orgasm

Another Eastern philosophy that can have a highly positive effect on your sex life is Daoism. Here, the woman is in control and the point of the slow build-up is a full body orgasm. This is an orgasm that isn't just confined to the genital area – it can suffuse your whole body , travelling round your legs, back up through your stomach and bursting from the top of your

> **TIP**
>
> If he massages the hollow between the tendon and the ankle bone, on both sides, it releases blocked kidney energy that leads to sexual inhibition. Massage here restores lost kidney energy, and arouses both of you.

head in a shower of spangles, leaving you limp and comatose with post-pleasure exhaustion. Or something like that, at any rate. Some women describe it as a tidal wave they're surfing, while still others find it such an emotional release they end up in tears.

There are various ways to arrive at this marvellous place. Daoism teaches many similar methods to tantra, with a few differences – the focus is on the genitals, and 'vaginal' and 'testicular' breathing – I know, I know, but stick with it.

First, release your Chi by slapping very lightly on your face, chest and legs – all over, in fact, to awaken your energy channels.

Rotate your hips, to get the energy flowing round your body, and make a 'shhhh' sound, to get rid of tension – come on, it's not that bad, singing teachers make you do this kind of thing. Well, some do.

The men, meanwhile, are rubbing their perineums (should that be 'perinea'?) and pulling on their penises while bending over and sticking their tongues out. Apparently the longer the tongue, the longer the penis, though that may just be something that Daoist teachers say to excuse their pupils looking like complete tools in front of each other.

Women now need to focus on their 'vaginal breathing', which means pulling energy towards their genitals, using deep breathing and concurrent clenching and releasing of the vaginal muscles. Concentrate on your outer labia, and pull inwards towards your inner labia, taking a short 'sip' of breath with each contraction. Do the same with your anus and perineum, for several repetitions. By 'breathing' this way, you can hold back each time your orgasm seems imminent – take your breath, clench, and as the feeling ebbs and comes back stronger, by the time you finally let it happen you may well have built yourself up to a full body orgasm – you'll know if you have, don't worry.

Ancient sexual wisdom suggests that the first, clitoral orgasm is merely the warm-up act – and that once she's come, she's primed and ready for a more intense, vaginal orgasm. The first orgasm dispels fear – just think of how relaxed you feel when you've come – and it allows her to embrace the full sexual experience with her partner afterwards.

Men have an equivalent method – 'testicle' breathing relies, again, on him taking his breaths and squeezing his testicles, anus and perineum in a short series of clenches to hold off orgasm, similar to tantric sex. This method does rely on exceptional control and patience from both partners, however, and if it gets too difficult, just get the vibrator out.

It is theoretically possible to experience a 'spiritual' orgasm from the shared mouth-breathing, while you're sitting on his lap, with your legs clasped behind him, and his legs crossed so you're as bodily close as it's

TIP

To help train your vaginal muscles to a peak of efficiency, you can either keep having babies, or do it the easy way. Start by inserting a biggish vibrator, and holding that in there – then progress through courgettes, bananas, small carrots, finally achieving the muscle control required to hold an object as thin as a pencil. Though if that's his penis, you may have a problem.

possible to be. This feels a little like the effects of Reiki healing, which also works on the chakras.

aphrodisiacs

To prepare for your nights of tantric/Taoist lovin', you may want to go the whole way and prepare a feast of aphrodisiacs to get both of you suitably worked up. But don't overeat, or you'll end up groaning with indigestion, rather than passion. Useful ingredients for your passion-stimulating meal include the following:

- anchovies
- caviar
- honey

- artichokes
- champagne
- salmon

- steak
- ginger
- vanilla

But of course, not all at once, because then you would be sick without a doubt. Most contain either stamina-boosting or stimulating chemicals – but if you don't want to have an aphrodisiac blow-out, stick with champagne, that's my advice.

yin & yang

The Chinese believe that men and women have different energies – Yin is female, and Yang is male – and that each one has different qualities to bring to life – and sex. Yang energy is dynamic, straightforward and immediate, whereas Yin energy is gentle, receptive and slower-paced. But mingling the two creates a perfect whole, of course. Suggestions for pre-sex mingling of energies – or foreplay, in other words – include the

> **TIP**
>
> If you really want to try and come during intercourse, one tip is for him to start by just barely inserting the head of his penis. He goes in and out for a few minutes, then goes in another half-inch, in and out for a few minutes ... keep going, half an inch at a time, until he's fully in – at which point you may or may not experience a mind-blowing, earth-shattering orgasm. It takes a lot of restraint for him to manage this, but if he does, it may well pay off, big time.

reminder that each partner doesn't necessarily want to receive exactly what they're giving, due to their different needs and energies. Yang is expected to give appropriately – which may mean responding to her needs very differently from how she responds to his own needs. While variety is required in foreplay, the ancient texts make it clear that if there are certain elements of foreplay that your partner loves, it's pointless to cut them out altogether just to be 'interesting'.

It's also vital to use all of the senses. In Chinese medicine, each sense corresponds to a certain orgasm – ears with kidneys, tongue with heart, lips with spleen, lungs with nose, and eyes with liver – so stimulating a particular sense helps Chi to flow from that organ, and theoretically balances your body's energies. Of course, that may strike you as a pile of pants, but the point of the exercise remains – that using all five senses massively enhances your sexual experience. Keep the room light, so you can see each other's bodies, and listen to your partner breathing, or gasping, which can be highly erotic. Touch, smell and taste are essential to good sex – scent particularly is the sense most directly connected to our emotional responses (which is why when you smell chalk, you're instantly transported

Some couples find it helpful to designate certain names to their genitals – purely because saying 'can you touch me down there,' or even 'now grab my cock' sounds either clinical or way too porn. The names you choose are entirely down to personal preference, whether calling his penis Mr Wibbly does it for you, or you actually prefer to use the old 'jade stalk' Chinese favourites. He might wish to call your bits 'Lady Jane' in the manner of D.H. Lawrence – or he might find 'Pussy' works just as well. Whatever you decide, just don't tell anyone else – they're sure to find it nauseating …

back to the classroom with all its attendant feelings). Humans secrete pheromones, too, which are chemical 'messengers' that arouse the opposite sex, which is why fresh (though not day-old) sweat can be such a turn on.

It's also recommended that you involve your whole body – which isn't as easy as it sounds, because most sexual activity tends to focus on the face, breasts and genitals – because integrating the whole of both your bodies invigorates sexual energy in both of you.

oral sex

The spiritual version of oral sex isn't that different from the ordinary version. But much to his delight, it's recommended that you swallow when he comes. Possibly all the writers of ancient Chinese texts were men, with an eye to the main chance – but still, as far as they were concerned, semen was a life force that heals all manner of ills (so when your partner insists that it 'cures sore throats' he may not be lying quite as much as he thinks he is). In fact, emperors allegedly used to collect the semen of younger men, mix it with herbs, and drink it in a bid to prolong their lives. And they did used to live quite a long time … but what a price to pay.

Oral sex, however, is considered the second most powerful way of transferring Chi between you – no prizes for guessing the first most powerful. The more Chi that flows between you, the more unified you get, and the more strengthened by each other's qualities.

Going down on a man puts him in a more 'yin' receptive position, too, and helps him to be more vulnerable and empathetic to the female position. Because the traditional dominant/vulnerable roles are swapped round when you go down on him, you'll have Chi flying about like nobody's business – so if it all gets uncomfortable, just give a little, without the pressure of making him come – you can always use your hand instead, or go on to have sex.

Him going down on you – or 'drinking from the jade fountain,' which sounds a great deal nicer – is also supposed to offer vital health-giving properties. Oral sex is probably the likeliest way a woman will orgasm, too, partly because you can relax without worrying about him and the urgent needs of his jade stalk.

emotional release

Spiritual sex is highly powerful – even if you don't buy into all the Chi business, having this sort of physical and emotional connection with another person opens up dormant areas of feeling, and it's not unusual to burst into tears. If this happens – to you or him – just cuddle each other. You don't need to get into a whole discussion about 'oh, I see, now you're in tears, I thought you were having fun …' unless they genuinely are crying because you had a row or the boss was mean. Otherwise, it's just about unleashing pent-up emotion, so let it happen, and resume what you were doing when everybody calms down.

how to discuss sex

Talking about sex is fraught with problems. Sexuality is such an intimate, vulnerable part of us that actually expressing any negative feelings regarding your, or your partner's, performance can end in a battle that makes *Star Wars* look like a playground fight.

It's always easier to discuss sex outside of the bedroom – once you're halfway through undressing each other, you suddenly piping up, 'you know when you do that thing with your mouth? I don't like it' will serve as something of a dampener. Being naked also makes you more vulnerable – so talking with clothes on, over a glass of wine one evening, places less pressure on you. Don't, however, sit opposite each other at the kitchen table, overhead light glaring down – he'll expect you to state the date and time into a tape recorder before you begin.

Talk around the subject before you get onto it. Talking about intimacy, or how much time you spend together – in, obviously, a non-judgmental and supportive way – can lead naturally onto sex. Whereas saying, 'right, I'm glad you're back; now, about the way you treat my clitoris,' is perhaps not the ideal way to approach it.

When you do get around to it, instigate a discussion about what you like in bed – without ever criticising things they've done in the past, of course. If that all feels way too confrontational, write him a letter suggesting all the things you could do to each other. Don't forget to mention things you might do to him, though.

spiritual intercourse

The positions remain more or less the same – the only difference is in the names. 'The dragon turns' sounds better than 'missionary,' and 'treading tigers' is more romantic than 'doggy style' – but it still means the same thing. The bit that counts, however, is 'transition,' from foreplay to inter-course, and for him, suggestions include not always entering you in the same way – sometimes he should thrust in hard, other times tease your clitoris with the tip of his penis before pushing in just a little way. Or he can enter you just two inches or so, then pull out and rub himself on your labia, before re-entering. Then he could enter you fast and suddenly, pull back, pause, and hover before surprising you by plunging straight back in.

If you're wet enough – or our old pal KY is available – he can enter you very, very slowly indeed, a centimetre at a time. This feels amazing for him, and builds up your anticipation to fever pitch. Don't keep it all at this pace, though – you might fall asleep.

He can even enter from a new angle – slightly to one side presses on normally untouched areas of your vaginal wall, and may result in all kinds of excitement. Pulling your vulva apart as he enters is also a new kind of thrill, because it exposes your clitoris and the surrounding nerves to much more stimulation than normal.

If he really wants to tease you, he can push at your vaginal entrance – without going any further. After a few pushes, you'll be begging him to enter – and let's face it, he's doesn't have that much self control, even if he is a Taoist master …

Transition suggestions for you include varying the tension of your vaginal muscles, again, by squeezing your PC. Contract as he enters, then release – or vice versa. This is easiest done lying on your back.

> **TIP**
>
> While it's fine to go along with a bit of action when you're not really in the mood, in the hope that it'll get you going, it's a different thing entirely to be sexually dishonest. If you're faking orgasms, or pretending to enjoy what he's doing when really you're screaming with internal boredom – don't do it. Just tell him the truth, as kindly as you can – and show him what he could be doing differently. Almost everyone wants to make their partner happy and satisfied in bed – so you owe each other the chance to do that. If all it takes is a simple adjustment of the finger or tongue, then surely it's better to find a way of saying so? Communication is the key to satisfying sex – and without it, all the sex tips in the world won't work.

Altering the angle of your legs also helps – if you put both feet on one of his shoulders, for instance, he can enter you slowly from a new position. Use your hands, too, against his hips, so you're controlling the depth of penetration – then suddenly move them so he thrusts into you unexpectedly for him. Also be aware that sometimes your genitals are arranged in a manner that means they don't fit together perfectly – he might have a long penis and you've got a short vagina, or your clitoris may be too high to be stimulated by his groin when he thrusts. This isn't necessarily a problem, but it is worth being aware of, because then you can rectify it. If you assume that everyone's built the same, you'll feel like it's someone's fault. It isn't – it may just mean you have to find a new way of doing things, to ensure your sexual fire burns as brightly as possible, for as long as possible.